Women's Health: A Resource Guide

Edited by
Pamela S. Dickerson, PhD, RN, BC

Oncology Nursing Society
Pittsburgh, Pennsylvania

BP45

ONS Publishing Division
Publisher: Leonard Mafrica, MBA, CAE
Director of Commercial Publishing: Barbara Sigler, RN, MNEd
Production Manager: Lisa M. George, BA
Technical Editor: Dorothy Mayernik, RN, MSN
Staff Editor: Lori Wilson, BA
Copy Editor: Amy Nicoletti, BA
Graphic Designer: Dany Sjoen

Women's Health: A Resource Guide for Nurses

Library of Congress Control Number: 2006928772

ISBN-13: 978-1-890504-61-8
ISBN-10: 1-890504-61-0

Publisher's Note
This book is published by the Oncology Nursing Society (ONS). ONS neither represents nor guarantees that the practices described herein will, if followed, ensure safe and effective patient care. The recommendations contained in this book reflect ONS's judgment regarding the state of general knowledge and practice in the field as of the date of publication. The recommendations may not be appropriate for use in all circumstances. Those who use this book should make their own determinations regarding specific safe and appropriate patient-care practices, taking into account the personnel, equipment, and practices available at the hospital or other facility at which they are located. The editors and publisher cannot be held responsible for any liability incurred as a consequence from the use or application of any of the contents of this book. Figures and tables are used as examples only. They are not meant to be all-inclusive, nor do they represent endorsement of any particular institution by ONS. Mention of specific products and opinions related to those products do not indicate or imply endorsement by ONS.

ONS publications are originally published in English. Permission has been granted by the ONS Board of Directors for foreign translation. (Individual tables and figures that are reprinted or adapted require additional permission from the original source.) However, because translations from English may not always be accurate or precise, ONS disclaims any responsibility for inaccuracies in words or meaning that may occur as a result of the translation. Readers relying on precise information should check the original English version.

Printed in the United States of America

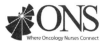

Oncology Nursing Society
Integrity • Innovation • Stewardship • Advocacy • Excellence • Inclusiveness

2/25/08

Contributors

Editor

Pamela S. Dickerson, PhD, RN, BC
President
PRN Continuing Education
Westerville, Ohio
Chapter 24. Relationship Transitions

Authors

Janet Akers, MSN, RN, CEN
In memorium
Chapter 10. Sexually Transmitted Infections;
Chapter 14. Domestic Violence

Myrna L. Armstrong, RN, EdD, FAAN
Professor, School of Nursing
Texas Tech University Health Sciences
  Center
TTU at Highland Lakes
Marble Falls, Texas
Chapter 11. Body Art: Tattooing, Body Piercing,
and Cosmetic Tattooing

Diana Fullen Bowers, PhD, RD, LD
Clinical Specialist/HomeReach, Inc.
OhioHealth
Columbus, Ohio
Chapter 16. Nutrition for Health Promotion;
Chapter 18. Herbals and Botanicals

Graham A. Colditz, MD, DrPH
Professor of Medicine
Harvard Medical School
Boston, Massachusetts
Chapter 21. Nurses' Health Study Update

Janis A. Cruce, MSN, RN, CS, FNP
Women Veterans Program Manager
Department of Veterans Affairs
VA Pacific Islands Health Care Systems
Honolulu, Hawaii
Chapter 17. Hormone Replacement Therapy;
Chapter 20. Health Screening and Monitoring

Kelly J. Damman, RN, OCN®
Lung Health Nurse
OhioHealth–Cancer Care Riverside
  Methodist Hospital
Columbus, Ohio
Chapter 5. Lung Cancer

Lynn Dobb, MA
Education Manager
Central Ohio Area Agency on Aging
Columbus, Ohio
Chapter 26. Adult Children and Aging Parents

Lisa Durham, MSW, LISW
Community Education and Outreach
  Director
Central Ohio Area Agency on Aging
Columbus, Ohio
Chapter 26. Adult Children and Aging Parents

LeaRae Galarowicz, MS, RN, BC
Clinical Professor and Manager,
  Continuing Nursing Education
School of Nursing
University of Wisconsin–Madison
Madison, Wisconsin
Chapter 23. Using Time Effectively

Dorothy J. Hall, MS, RN, CNS
Mental Health Nurse Consultant
Westerville, Ohio
Chapter 9. Depression

Ellen Homlong, RD, LD, CDE
Clinical and Patient Service Manager
HDS Services/Samaritan Hospital
Ashland, Ohio
Chapter 13. Eating Disorders

Carolen Koleszar, BSN, RN
Naturopath
Health for Everyone, Inc.
New Albany, Ohio
Chapter 19. Naturopathic Care

Lori Kondas, BA, RRT, CPFT, AE-C
Vice President, Program Services
American Lung Association® of Ohio
Independence, Ohio
Chapter 12. Smoking and Smoking Cessation

Leona Lipari Lee, MA, RN
Retired
Bay St. Louis, Missouri
Chapter 25. Surviving Menopause

Ruth Leslie, RN, CD
Regional Liaison Person
Peer Assistance Program for Nurses
Director of Nursing
Glenbeigh Hospital and Outpatient
  Facility
Rock Creek, Ohio
Chapter 15. Chemical Dependency

Joanne Lester, MSN, RNC, CNP,
  AOCN®
Oncology Nurse Practitioner
James Cancer Hospital & Solove Research
  Institute
Ohio State University
Columbus, Ohio
Chapter 3. Breast Health and Breast Cancer

Jacqueline M. Loversidge, MS, RN, C
Assistant Professor and Director
Nursing Accelerated Program
Capital University
Columbus, Ohio
Chapter 22. Stress Management

Betsy McClung, MN, RN
Associate Director
Oregon Osteoporosis Center
Portland, Oregon
Chapter 2. Osteoporosis

Sarah McGrew, BSN
National Trainer for the Arthritis
  Foundation
Manager of Clinical and Community
  Experiences
College of Osteopathic Medicine
Ohio University
Athens, Ohio
Chapter 6. Fibromyalgia Syndrome

Shirlien Metersky, MSN, RN, CCRN
CCU Educator
Grant Medical Center
Columbus, Ohio
Chapter 1. Heart Health

Zandra Ohri, MA, MS, RN
Director, Nursing Education and Peer
  Assistance Program for Nurses
Ohio Nurses Association
Columbus, Ohio
Chapter 15. Chemical Dependency

Christine A. Price, PhD, CFLE
Assistant Professor
Family and Child Studies Department
Montclair State University
Montclair, New Jersey
Chapter 27. Retirement Issues

Lee Ann Ruess, MS, RN, CCRN, CNS,
  APRN,BC
Clinical Faculty
College of Nursing
Ohio State University
Columbus, Ohio
Chapter 8. Fertility Challenges

Doreen A. White, BSN, RN, CWOCN
Wound, Ostomy, and Continence Nurse
  Consultant
Springfield, Ohio
Chapter 7. Urinary Incontinence

Marcella Williams, MS, RN, AOCN®
Scientific Writer
OES Division, Oncology Nursing Society
Pittsburgh, Pennsylvania
Chapter 4. Gynecologic Cancers

Table of Contents

Preface

Welcome to *Women's Health: A Resource Guide for Nurses*. Women's health is a fascinating topic—both because of the emerging research on women's issues and because, in a predominantly female profession, nurses need to be knowledgeable about issues that affect themselves and their female patients. This book is written with both of those perspectives in mind. The book was developed as a resource for nurses to provide up-to-date information as a tool for patient teaching. Females in the nursing profession also may find it useful for self-education.

Because this is a book about women, the word "her" is used as a primary reference pronoun. This does not mean that information does not or could not apply to men. Most questions reflect the feminine viewpoint. However, the more universal pronouns (his or her) are used when appropriate to the question.

As I have worked with the authors of this book, I have continually been amazed by the areas of connection between chapters. For example, the theme of smoking cessation carries through many of the chapters, although a specific chapter provides detailed information about stopping smoking. Many "connections" will become apparent as you explore the chapters. This exemplifies the fact that humans really are holistic beings, with integrated body systems and life functions.

The book is written based on current information, research findings, and therapeutic interventions. When medications are mentioned, drug names are used as examples and are not meant to be all-inclusive or specific recommendations. Always consult your own healthcare provider for information specific to your individual situation, and encourage patients to do the same. Research is continuing at a rapid pace, so it is important that all healthcare professionals keep up with emerging changes. I hope that this text will aid you in caring for your female patients.

Chapter 1

Heart Health

Shirlien Metersky, MSN, RN, CCRN

Background/Significance

Q 1.1 **What does the term "cardiovascular disease" refer to?**

"Cardiovascular disease" refers to diseases of the heart and blood vessels. These include heart attacks, high blood pressure, coronary heart disease, disease in the blood vessels of the legs, and stroke. For the purposes of this chapter, "cardiovascular disease" will be referred to as "heart disease" unless otherwise noted.

Q 1.2 **What does "family history" of heart disease mean?**

A "family history" of heart disease refers to having a father or brother who had a heart attack before age 55 or a mother or sister who had a heart attack before age 65.

Q 1.3 **What is the prevalence of heart disease in women compared to other causes of death?**

Heart disease is the leading cause of death for American women. In the United States, more women die of heart disease than the next 10 causes of death combined. Nearly twice as many women die of heart disease and stroke than of *all* forms of cancer (Mosca, Ferris, Fabunmi, & Robertson, 2004). One in every 2 women will die of heart disease, whereas 1 in 27 women will die of breast cancer. Heart disease is not a "guy thing." More women than men die of heart disease. In 2002, 493,623 women died of heart disease compared to 433,825 men (American Heart Association [AHA], 2005g). Although these statistics are frightening, heart disease is largely preventable. Taking control of heart risk factors and adopting heart-healthy habits can greatly decrease the development and progression of heart disease.

Q 1.4   Is the prognosis after having a heart attack better in men or women?

Women who present with symptoms of a heart attack are less likely to be admitted to the hospital or may get a different level of treatment because women's symptoms often are unrecognized or misdiagnosed. Once women have been diagnosed with a heart attack, their prognosis is worse. More women than men die within one year of having a heart attack. Women also are more likely than men to have a stroke or a second heart attack within six years after having an initial heart attack (National Coalition for Women with Heart Disease, 2005).

Q 1.5   Which women are at the highest risk for heart attack and stroke?

African American women have the highest risk of having a heart attack or stroke in comparison to females of other ethnic groups. African American women develop heart disease at an earlier age, have a higher incidence of heart risk factors such as high blood pressure, diabetes, and obesity, and have a higher death rate from heart disease. Financial status, cultural beliefs, family behaviors, and access to health care may be reasons for a higher incidence of heart disease for African American women (AHA, 2005c).

Risk Factors

Q 1.6   What should be included with a heart risk assessment and screening?

Many women are interested in talking to their healthcare providers about heart disease and ways to prevent it. However, the majority of women never reach the point of having this discussion. All women should ask their healthcare providers to talk with them about their heart risk factors. Medical professionals should perform an assessment of patients' heart risk factors at every visit, which should include the following considerations (Faucher, Stewart-Fahs, Fleschler, Goss, & Moody, 2001).
• Tobacco use or exposure to secondhand smoke
• Weight
• Diet and nutrition
• Physical activity
• Blood pressure
• Family history of heart disease

- Age
- Racial, ethnic, cultural, and socioeconomic factors
- Stress levels and depression

Periodic screening for heart disease also should include (Faucher et al., 2001)

- Lipid panel profile every five years after age 20 (earlier or more frequent testing may be needed if abnormal results or multiple risk factors are present)
- Diabetes testing every three years after age 45 (earlier or more frequent testing should be performed if any of the following diabetes risk factors are present: family history of diabetes, obesity, physical inactivity, high blood pressure, high cholesterol levels, delivery of a baby weighing more than nine pounds, polycystic ovary syndrome, or African American, Hispanic, Native American, Asian American, or Pacific Islander ethnicity).

1.7   Does the risk of heart disease increase after menopause?

Women's risk of heart disease increases significantly after menopause. Women often do not show signs of heart disease until about 10 years later than men. As women age, their risk of heart disease and stroke begins to gradually rise. Although younger men have more heart attacks than women, by age 75, women and men are equal in their chances of having a heart attack (Faucher et al., 2001). One thing to note is that if menopause is caused by surgery to remove the uterus and ovaries, the risk of heart disease rises sharply, whereas if menopause occurs naturally, the risk of heart disease rises more slowly (AHA, 2005d).

1.8   Which heart risk factors can women control?

Choosing one's parents, race, and age are risk factors that women cannot control. The good news is that people *can* control many other heart risk factors. Risk factors that women have control over include smoking, high blood pressure, elevated cholesterol levels, physical inactivity, overweight and obesity, and diabetes. Gaining control over these risk factors will greatly reduce one's risk of developing heart disease.

1.9   How does having diabetes affect my risk of heart disease?

The incidence of diabetes has been rising steadily in the United States, with women accounting for more than half of all adults with the disease. Heart disease death rates for diabetics are two to four times higher than for adults without diabetes, and diabetics are at a much higher risk of having a stroke (AHA, 2005b). Diabetics often have high blood pressure and cholesterol levels and are overweight. These factors increase their risk of heart disease even more. The good news is that people can control diabetes and lower their risk of heart disease by choosing a healthy diet, getting exercise, and maintaining a healthy weight.

Q 1.10   Is where excess weight is "carried" important as a heart risk factor in women?

Carrying an excess amount of fat, especially around the waist, increases the risk of developing heart disease. In other words, being "apple-shaped" is worse than being "pear-shaped." A woman's waist should measure less than 35 inches (Faucher et al., 2001).

Q 1.11   I am overweight. How will losing weight help to reduce my risk of heart disease?

One-third of American women are obese, and the number keeps rising (American Stroke Association/AHA, 2005). A woman who carries excess weight is at a higher risk for developing health problems such as high blood pressure, high cholesterol levels, heart disease, and stroke. Being overweight also makes diabetes more likely to develop. Imagine carrying a 35-pound box up a flight of stairs. Most people would be short of breath, and their hearts would be beating faster. If people are carrying that same amount of extra weight on their bodies, then their hearts are working too hard. Losing as little as 7–15 pounds can make a difference in people's heart health, and they can better manage blood pressure, cholesterol levels, and diabetes. If people are serious about losing weight, they will be more successful if they diet and exercise. Diet or exercise alone is not as effective in weight reduction.

Q 1.12   How is hypertension now defined?

"Hypertension" is defined as a blood pressure reading of 140/90 or greater that stays high for an extended period of time. Table 1-1 describes blood pressure classifications with recommended follow-up time frames (National Heart, Lung, and Blood Institute, 2003). High blood pressure may not have any symptoms—the only way to know whether a person has high blood pressure is to measure it. One

Table 1-1. Blood Pressure Classifications With Recommended Follow-Up

Category	Systolic Reading		Diastolic Reading	Recommended Follow-Up
Normal	< 120	And	Less than 80	Recheck in two years.
Prehypertension	120–139	Or	85–89	Recheck in one year.
Hypertension				
• Stage 1	140–159	Or	90–99	Confirm within two months.
• Stage 2	≥ 160	Or	≥ 100	Evaluate within one month.
				Evaluate and treat immediately or within one week for blood pressure > 180/110.

Note. Based on information from National Heart, Lung, and Blood Institute, 2003.

out of 4 adults has high blood pressure and does not even know it, and only 1 in 4 adults being treated with medicine for high blood pressure has his or her blood pressure under control.

1.13   What is a lipid panel, and what do the values mean?

A lipid panel looks at both the total cholesterol level and at the individual elements. Two main types of cholesterol exist. Low-density lipoprotein (LDL) is known as the "bad" cholesterol because too much LDL causes a buildup in arteries that makes blood flow more difficult. High-density lipoprotein (HDL) is known as the "good" cholesterol because it helps to clear out excess cholesterol and reduces the buildup of LDL. Higher levels of HDL decrease the risk of heart disease. An easy way to remember the difference between LDL and HDL is that a person wants low LDL and high HDL. Recommendations for optimal LDL values are based on risk categories for heart disease. Table 1-2 reviews the risk categories that modify LDL goals.

In addition, a lipid panel assesses triglyceride levels. High triglyceride levels also are present in people with heart disease. Table 1-3 shows the optimal values for lipid panel numbers.

Table 1-2. Risk Categories That Modify Low-Density Lipoprotein (LDL) Cholesterol Goals

Risk Category	LDL Cholesterol Goal
CHD', at very high risk	< 70
CHD and CHD risk equivalents"	< 100
Multiple (2+) risk factors"'	< 130
Zero to one risk factor	< 160

'CHD (coronary heart disease)—includes history of heart attack, unstable or stable angina, or coronary artery procedure (angioplasty or bypass surgery)
"CHD risk equivalent—includes peripheral arterial disease, abdominal aortic aneurysm, carotid artery disease, and diabetes
"'Risk factors—include tobacco use, hypertension (blood pressure > 140/90 or on antihypertensive medication), low high-density lipoprotein cholesterol (< 40), family history of premature CHD, and age (men ≥ 45 years and women ≥ 55 years)

Note. Based on information from Grundy et al., 2004.

Table 1-3. Optimal Values for Lipid Panel Numbers

Panel	Level
Lipids	
Total cholesterol	< 200
Low-density lipoprotein cholesterol	< 100 = Optimal
	100–129 = Near optimal
	130–159 = Borderline high
High-density lipoprotein cholesterol	> 50 for women (> 40 for men)
Triglycerides	< 150

Note. Based on information from Grundy et al., 2004.

Q 1.14   Is it true that smoking is the number-one preventable heart risk?

Yes, smoking is the number-one preventable heart risk (Faucher et al., 2001). No matter how old a person is or how long he or she has smoked, quitting will greatly reduce his or her chances of developing heart disease. In the first year alone after stopping smoking, the risk of heart disease is cut in half. Within 10–15 years, the risk drops to the same risk level as someone who has never smoked (AHA, 2005a). It may take several tries for smokers to quit completely and permanently. Help from a healthcare provider and follow-up support will increase one's chance of being successful in quitting.

Q 1.15   What types of exercise are best?

Vigorous activities such as jogging, brisk walking, bicycling, or swimming for 30 minutes for at least four days a week are recommended. If a person is not an exercise fanatic, low- to moderate-level activities such as walking, yard work, or housework for 30 minutes on most days are recommended. If people do not have 30 continuous minutes to carve out of their day, they can try three 10-minute or two 15-minute periods (AHA, 2005f). The important thing is to get up and get moving: Active women have a 50% reduction in heart risk (Faucher et al., 2001).

Q 1.16   Healthcare providers recommend reaching and sustaining a target heart rate while exercising. How is a target heart rate calculated?

People can use target heart rates to measure their fitness level and to evaluate their progress in a fitness program. The target heart rate should be 50%–75% of an individual's maximum heart rate. A person's maximum heart rate is approximately 220 minus the person's age (AHA, 2005e).

Taking one's pulse while exercising can be a challenge. One method to monitor progress during moderate activities like walking is to use the "conversational" pacing method. If people can walk and have a conversation, then they are not working too hard. If they can sing while exercising, then they are not working hard enough. If people cannot talk while exercising because of difficulty breathing, then they are working too hard.

Treatment

Q 1.17   Does taking hormone replacement therapy (HRT) provide protection against heart disease?

As menopause approaches, a woman's risk of heart disease increases and continues to increase as she ages. Some sources correlate this increased risk to lower estrogen levels. If that is the case, it would make sense that HRT would add some protection against heart disease. However, recent studies do not confirm the benefit of HRT for the sole purpose of protection against heart disease. In fact, women need to be aware of extra heart disease risks associated with the use of HRT. HRT is not a treatment for heart disease (AHA, 2005d).

Q 1.18   Why is it harder to diagnose a heart attack in women?

Classic symptoms of a heart attack include pain or pressure in the middle of the chest that may spread to the neck, shoulders, or arms. Women usually present with less common warning signs of heart attack, such as abdominal pain, nausea and/or vomiting, dizziness, shortness of breath, unexplained anxiety, weakness or fatigue, or a cold sweat. Such vague symptoms make it difficult to diagnose a heart attack quickly in women. In fact, many women receive misdiagnoses or do not even seek medical help because they think symptoms are just indigestion or "the flu" and that they will pass (Rosenfeld, 2001).

Q 1.19   Are women treated differently than men in the management of heart disease?

Unfortunately, women do tend to receive different treatment than men. Healthcare professionals handle the management of heart disease from primary prevention through diagnosis, treatment, and follow-up care differently with women. Physicians are less likely to screen women for heart risk factors, or they may perceive women's risk as low. Therefore, they underestimate women's heart risk and miss opportunities to prevent heart disease (Mosca et al., 2005). Because a woman's warning signs of heart attack may be vague, healthcare providers often dismiss or overlook these symptoms. Medical professionals refer women less often or later than men for diagnostic heart catheterizations. Even when women present with heart attack symptoms and multiple risk factors, they are less likely to receive *early* treatment to open blocked coronary arteries, such as "clot-busting" drugs, balloon dilatation, or bypass surgery. Women also are less likely to be enrolled into cardiac rehabilitation programs after a heart attack or bypass surgery (Rosenfeld, 2001).

Q 1.20   Are there diagnostic tests for heart disease that are preferred for women?

The exercise stress test produces more false positives in women than in men. Therefore, if a woman has a positive test, the physician may dismiss the result as an error and not pursue the possibility of the presence of heart disease. Imaging stress testing is more sensitive than exercise stress testing ("Testing and Diagnosis," 2005). A more reliable diagnostic test is a stress echocardiogram (ultrasound of the heart) or a stress nuclear imaging test, which maps the heart to look for areas that are not receiving an adequate blood supply.

Q 1.21   Are antioxidants and vitamins helpful in the prevention of heart disease?

Nutritional supplementation for the prevention or reduction of heart disease is a controversial subject. Some antioxidants or vitamins are thought to be helpful, but not enough evidence exists to support their use in the prevention or treatment of heart disease (Mayo Clinic, 2006). Antioxidants are thought to reduce the risk of heart disease because they may lower the amount of LDL (bad) cholesterol. Examples of antioxidants are vitamin C, vitamin E, and beta-carotene. However, recent studies on vitamin E suggest that vitamin E in amounts greater than 400 IU (international units) per day may increase the risk of death. Taking nutritional supplements should never replace eating a heart-healthy diet rich in fruits and vegetables and low in saturated fat. Taking control over other heart risk factors such as smoking and high blood pressure will have more benefit than nutritional supplements.

Q 1.22   What should I do if I think I am having a heart attack?

A person should call 911 if experiencing the warning signs of a heart attack. Remember that these can include classic chest discomfort or less common warning signs, such as abdominal pain, sweating, or shortness of breath. The person should stop whatever activity he or she is doing, and rest. Take an aspirin if readily available (not acetaminophen or a nonsteroidal anti-inflammatory drug). The average person waits three to four hours before seeking medical attention, and women tend to delay longer than men. The more time that is wasted, the more the heart will be damaged.

References

American Heart Association. (2005a). *Cigarette smoking and cardiovascular diseases.* Retrieved September 2, 2005, from http://www.americanheart.org/presenter.jhtml?identifier=4545
American Heart Association. (2005b). *Facts about women's heart disease and stroke risk factors.* Retrieved September 2, 2005, from http://www.americanheart.org/presenter.jhtml?identifier=4786

American Heart Association. (2005c). *Heart disease and stroke facts about African-American women*. Retrieved September 2, 2005, from http://www.americanheart.org/downloadable/heartsmart/1082152750133GRFWFactsaboutA-AWomenandCVD.doc

American Heart Association. (2005d). *Menopause and the risk of heart disease and stroke*. Retrieved September 2, 2005, from http://www.americanheart.org/presenter.jhtml?identifier=1024

American Heart Association. (2005e). *Target heart rates*. Retrieved September 2, 2005, from http://www.americanheart.org/presenter.jhtml?identifier=4736

American Heart Association. (2005f). *Ten questions a woman should ask her healthcare provider*. Retrieved September 2, 2005, from http://www.americanheart.org/presenter.jhtml?identifier=2759

American Heart Association. (2005g). *Women and cardiovascular diseases—Statistics by the American Heart Association*. Retrieved June 1, 2005, from http://www.americanheart.org/downloadable/heart/1109000876764FS10WM05REV.DOC

American Stroke Association/American Heart Association. (2005). *A nation at risk: Obesity in the United States statistical sourcebook*. Retrieved September 2, 2005, from http://www.americanheart.org

Faucher, M.A., Stewart-Fahs, P., Fleschler, R., Goss, G.L., & Moody, K.B. (2001). *Evidence-based clinical practice guidelines. Cardiovascular health for women: Primary prevention*. Washington, DC: Association of Women's Health, Obstetric and Neonatal Nurses.

Grundy, S.M., Cleeman, J.I., Merz, C.N., Brewer, H.B., Jr., Clark, L.T., Hunninghake, D.B., et al. (2004). Implications of recent clinical trials for the NCEP Adult Treatment Panel III guidelines. *Circulation, 110*, 227–239.

Mayo Clinic. (2006, February). *Antioxidant supplements: Can they prevent heart disease?* Retrieved February 3, 2006, from http://www.mayoclinic.com/health/antioxidant-supplements/AN01147

Mosca, L., Ferris, A., Fabunmi, R., & Robertson, R.M. (2004). Tracking women's awareness of heart disease: An American Heart Association national study. *Circulation, 109*, 573–579.

Mosca, L., Linfante, A.H., Benjamin, E.J., Berra, K., Hayes, S.N., Walsh, B.W., et al. (2005). National study of physician awareness and adherence to cardiovascular disease prevention guidelines. *Circulation, 111*, 499–510.

National Coalition for Women with Heart Disease. (2005). *Women and heart disease fact sheet*. Retrieved June 1, 2005, from http://www.womenheart.org/information/women_and_heart_disease_fact_sheet.asp

National Heart, Lung, and Blood Institute. (2003, August). *Seventh report of the Joint National Committee on prevention, detection, evaluation, and treatment of high blood pressure* (NIH Publication No. 04-5230). Bethesda, MD: U.S. Department of Health and Human Services.

Rosenfeld, A.G. (2001). Women's risk of decision delay in acute myocardial infarction: Implications for research and practice. *AACN Clinical Issues, 12*, 29–39.

Testing and diagnosis. (2005). *Professional view, Heart Healthy Women*. Retrieved June 1, 2005, from http://www.hearthealthywomen.org/professionals/testing_diagnosis/stress_test_ecg.html

Resources

American Heart Association: www.americanheart.org

Association for Women's Health, Obstetric and Neonatal Nursing (AWHONN): www.awhonn.org

Mosca, L., Appel, L.J., Benjamin, E.J., Berra, K., Chandra-Strobos, N., Fabunmi, R.P., et al. (2004). Evidence-based guidelines for cardiovascular disease prevention in women. *Circulation, 109*, 672–693.

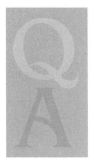

Chapter 2
Osteoporosis

Betsy McClung, MN, RN

Background

2.1 What is osteoporosis?

Osteoporosis has been defined as a systemic skeletal disease characterized by low bone mass and microarchitectural deterioration of bone tissue, which leads to enhanced bone fragility and a consequential increase in fracture risk ("Consensus Development Conference," 1991). The National Institutes of Health (2001) Consensus Statement on Osteoporosis expanded the earlier definition by describing osteoporosis as a skeletal disorder characterized by compromised bone strength.

Bone strength reflects the integration of two main features: bone mineral density (BMD) and bone quality. BMD is expressed as grams of mineral per area or volume. It is a function of how much bone was made during years of skeletal growth and how much bone subsequently may have been lost. "Bone quality" refers to architecture that is affected by bone turnover, damage accumulation such as microfractures, and mineralization. Currently, no accurate way exists to measure bone strength. BMD frequently serves as a proxy measure and accounts for approximately 70% of bone strength (Jergas & Genant, 1993).

2.2 What are the physical signs of osteoporosis?

Physical signs of osteoporosis include vertebral compression fracture; kyphosis (thoracic spinal curvature) and/or protruding abdomen; back pain, paraspinal muscle tenderness, and back fatigue; height loss greater than 1.5 inches; hip fracture; and wrist fracture.

Q __2.3__ **What is the most important goal of osteoporosis prevention and treatment strategies?**

The most important therapeutic goal is to prevent fractures, particularly fractures of the spine and hip. These fractures lead to severe complications that affect an individual's quality of life, morbidity, and mortality.

Q __2.4__ **What are the major risk factors for postmenopausal osteoporosis (low bone mass)?**

Key risk factors include estrogen deficiency, advanced age, personal history of fracture as an adult, family history of osteoporosis and/or spine or hip fracture, and small body frame or low body weight (less than 127 pounds) (Cummings et al., 1995).

Medical causes of osteoporosis include taking medications such as steroids or antiseizure medications or excessive use of thyroid hormone. Certain medical conditions including hyperparathyroidism or malabsorption also may contribute to low bone mass.

Diagnosis/Screening

Q __2.5__ **How is osteoporosis diagnosed?**

Healthcare professionals use radiographic evaluation to confirm the diagnosis of osteoporosis in a patient with spine fracture. Osteoporotic spine fracture results in a change in the shape of the vertebral body that can be seen on x-ray and can serve, to some extent, to evaluate the severity of osteoporosis. Variations in x-ray exposure, however, make x-ray evaluation unreliable in assessing the degree of low bone mass.

BMD testing is the most accurate technology used to make the diagnosis of osteoporosis in postmenopausal women. The important criterion for BMD testing is that the result will be of value in making treatment decisions. For example, BMD measurement has no role in healthy, estrogen-replete premenopausal women because the results would not influence patient management beyond any general recommendations that should be made regardless of their BMD values.

Q 2.6 I am postmenopausal. What guidelines are recommended for bone density testing?

Bone density testing is indicated for women who possess character-istics that are associated with low BMD. This includes all women 65 years of age and older regardless of risk factors and younger post-menopausal women with other risk factors. The most important of these risk factors are small body size (weight less than 127 pounds), history of fragility fracture in a first-degree relative, personal history of fracture as an adult, current smoking, use of oral corticosteroid therapy for more than three months, and x-ray evidence of low bone mass (National Osteoporosis Foundation, 2003).

Q 2.7 Why is central dual-energy x-ray absorptiometry (DEXA) of the spine and hip considered to be the gold standard for measuring BMD?

Central DEXA is the only test that can be used to make the diagnosis of osteoporosis and monitor BMD changes over time in response to therapy. The World Health Organization defines the central DEXA T score, –2.5, as the threshold for osteoporosis diagnosis (WHO Study Group, 1994). Healthcare professionals cannot use peripheral T scores of the heel, wrist, and finger for diagnosis because of marked differences in rates of age-related bone loss measured by different technologies in these sites. Peripheral T scores are not equivalent with central T scores of the spine and/or hip. In addition, peripheral sites are inadequate to monitor response to therapy because BMD in these sites changes minimally in response to antiresorptive therapy.

Medical professionals often advocate use of peripheral devices for screening rather than diagnosis. However, these tests often func-tion poorly in this role. A significant proportion of patients with or without osteoporosis receive misdiagnoses, leading to unnecessary anxiety and possibly inappropriate treatment.

Q 2.8 What is a T score?

The T score is the bone density value expressed as the number of standard deviations above (+) or below (–) the average value in young, healthy women between the ages of 20 and 30. Healthy, young women normally have T scores between –2 and +2. Postmenopausal women with values between –2 and –2.5 are said to have low BMD. These values do not necessarily mean that bone loss has occurred. These values may be the result of lower-than-average peak bone mass, perhaps as a consequence of genetics. T scores with a number lower than –2.5 are consistent with the diagnosis of osteoporosis.

Q   2.9   Does a T score value of –2 represent the same osteoporotic fracture risk in a 55-year-old woman as in a 70-year-old woman?

No. Age is a more important indicator of fracture probability than BMD. Thus, if two women, ages 50 and 70, have the same low BMD value, the older woman is more likely to have a fracture in the next five years because, in part, of the architectural changes that happen with aging bone.

Q   2.10   What are the objectives for assessing patients at risk for osteoporotic fracture?

- Confirm the correct diagnosis.
  - Although a history of back pain associated with kyphosis, height loss, and vertebral fracture in a postmenopausal woman may cause the clinician to suspect osteoporosis, a correct diagnosis is important. It is essential to rule out other causes of back pain, such as osteoarthritis, certain types of cancer, or degenerative disc disease.
- Identify contributing factors to low bone mass.
  - Nutrition (especially calcium and/or vitamin D deficiency)
  - Genetics (history of first-degree relative with nontraumatic fracture and/or diagnosed with osteoporosis)
  - Lifestyle (current smoking, excessive alcohol intake)
  - Medications known to cause bone loss (the most common is glucocorticoids)
  - History of fractures as an adult
  - Sex steroid deficiency
- Assess physical status.
  - Height measurement (maximum height versus current measurement)
    * Two-thirds of vertebral compression fractures are asymptomatic.
    * Height loss of more than 1.5 inches may suggest the presence of an undiagnosed fracture.
    * Having had one vertebral fracture greatly increases the risk of subsequent fractures.
    * Verify presence of suspected fracture(s) with spine radiograph.
  - Weight

– Evidence of kyphosis
– Muscle strength
– Vision
– Balance

Q 2.11 **What laboratory tests are used to identify patients with secondary causes of osteoporosis, such as calcium malabsorption, vitamin D deficiency, and hyperparathyroidism?**

Biochemical testing to identify causes of secondary osteoporosis may include
• Complete blood count
• Serum chemistries (calcium, phosphate, alkaline phosphatase, albumin, creatinine)
• 24-hour urinary calcium
• Secondary tests (25-OH vitamin D, parathyroid hormone [PTH], serum protein electrophoresis, thyroid-stimulating hormone, urinary cortisol)
• Biochemical markers of bone turnover.

Q 2.12 **When is it appropriate for a person to be referred to an osteoporosis specialist?**

Referral to an osteoporosis specialist is appropriate when the patient's clinical findings reveal complex secondary factors, such as the following (Hodgson et al., 2001).
• Osteoporosis that is unexpectedly severe or has unusual features at the time of initial assessment
• Very low BMD (a T score below –3.0 or a Z score below –2.0) (Note: A Z score is the number of standard deviations above or below the average value in an individual of the same age and gender.)
• Osteoporosis despite young age (premenopausal)
• Fractures despite borderline or normal BMD
• Fractures despite treatment
• Suspected or known condition that may underlie the osteoporosis (e.g., hyperthyroidism, hyperparathyroidism, Cushing syndrome, hypogonadism)
• Candidate for combination therapy
• Intolerance to approved therapies
• Failure to respond to treatment
• Low baseline BMD despite estrogen therapy
• Loss of BMD on serial DEXA studies while on osteoporosis drug therapy

Prevention/Treatment

Q 2.13   What is the recommended dietary allowance (RDA) for calcium intake in adult women and men?

The RDA for adults older than age 50 is a total of 1,200 mg of calcium per day. Vitamin D is necessary for optimal calcium absorption. The recommended vitamin D intake is 400 IU per day for adults age 51–70 and 600 IU for adults older than age 70 (Standing Committee on the Scientific Evaluation of Dietary Reference Intakes, 1997).

Q 2.14   What is a quick and easy way to estimate my daily dietary calcium intake?

Here is an easy formula for estimating individual daily calcium intake. First, assume that even a dairy-free (grains and vegetables) diet provides 300 mg of calcium. Then, add each dairy serving (approximately 300 mg of calcium for each 8-ounce glass of milk, carton of yogurt, or slice of cheese), any serving of calcium-fortified food, plus any calcium supplement. This formula determines the total calcium intake for the day (Endocrine Nurses Society, 2002).

Q 2.15   What are the most common types of calcium supplements?

The most common calcium salts are calcium carbonate and calcium citrate. People should take calcium carbonate with meals to aid absorption. It is inexpensive and is found in a wide range of doses, with or without vitamin D. It may cause constipation or gas, which people can manage by increasing fluid intake and physical activity. Calcium citrate does not need to be taken with meals. Calcium citrate supplements typically are more expensive than calcium carbonate and often require taking more tablets to get the same dose of elemental calcium. Regardless of the supplement, people should take no more than 600 mg of calcium at any one time.

Q 2.16   What are the approved pharmacologic therapies currently used to treat postmenopausal women diagnosed with osteoporosis to prevent fracture(s)?

The current therapies approved by the U.S. Food and Drug Administration for the treatment of osteoporosis include
• Bisphosphonates

- Alendronate (Fosamax®, Merck, Whitehouse Station, NJ): 10 mg every day or 70 mg once per week
- Risedronate (Actonel®, Procter & Gamble, Cincinnati, OH): 5 mg every day or 35 mg once per week
- Ibandronate (Boniva®, Roche Pharmaceuticals, Nutley, NJ): 2.5 mg every day or 150 mg once a month
- PTH (Forteo™, Eli Lilly, Indianapolis, IN): 20 mcg per day as subcutaneous injection
- Raloxifene (Evista®, Eli Lilly): 60 mg every day
- Calcitonin (Miacalcin®, Novartis, East Hanover, NJ) nasal spray: 200 IU every day.

Note: Combination drug therapy has not been adequately evaluated and should be reserved for patients in whom single-agent therapy has been shown to be ineffective.

Q 2.17 How do bisphosphonates work?

Bisphosphonates are a class of nonhormonal bone-specific compounds that inhibit bone resorption and prevent bone loss. Included in this class of drugs are alendronate (Fosamax), risedronate (Actonel), and ibandronate (Boniva). The drug binds to bone and decreases the activity of osteoclasts, the bone-dissolving cells. The result is inhibition of bone resorption, prevention of bone loss, and a 50%–60% reduction in the incidence of spine and non-spine fractures, including the hip (Harris et al., 1999; Liberman et al., 1995; Miller et al., 2004).

Q 2.18 How does Evista differ from Fosamax, Actonel, and Boniva?

Evista is a nonhormonal drug that has estrogen-like effects on the skeleton but blocks the estrogen effects in the breast and uterus. Treatment of women with postmenopausal osteoporosis for three years with Evista resulted in small increases in spine and hip BMD and reduced spine fractures by 30%–50%. Researchers observed no effect on non-spine fractures, including hip fractures (Ettinger et al., 1999). Healthcare professionals usually prescribe this drug to treat postmenopausal women at increased risk for spine fracture but whose risk for hip fracture is quite low.

Q 2.19 What is Forteo?

Forteo (teriparatide) is PTH, a protein hormone made by the parathyroid glands that regulates calcium and bone metabolism.

Q 2.20   How does Forteo differ from other treatments for osteoporosis?

The antiresorptive drugs (Fosamax, Actonel, and Evista) work by decreasing the activity of bone-dissolving cells and prevent the progression of bone loss rather than building new bone. PTH stimulates the activity of bone-building cells (osteoblasts), repairs damaged architecture, and thus improves the structure and strength of bone. Forteo increases BMD and reduces the risk of vertebral and nonvertebral fractures (Neer et al., 2001).

Q 2.21   Why does Forteo need to be given by injection?

Forteo is a protein hormone like insulin. If taken by mouth, it would be digested before it was absorbed.

Q 2.22   Why might Forteo be indicated for me?

Forteo is indicated for postmenopausal women with osteoporosis who are at very high fracture risk. These include women with a history of osteoporotic fracture(s), those who have multiple risk factors for fracture, or those who have failed or are intolerant of previous osteoporosis therapy.

Q 2.23   What is the most effective therapy for chronic back pain associated with osteoporotic vertebral fractures?

An effective therapy for chronic back pain is a consistent exercise program aimed at stretching and strengthening the paraspinal muscles. An experienced physical therapist can prescribe and monitor the exercise program and make adjustments according to the severity of the osteoporosis.

Q 2.24   I had a hip fracture. Should I be treated with an osteoporosis drug to prevent a second hip fracture?

Not all patients who suffer a hip fracture have osteoporosis. Independent clinical risk factors exist for falls and injuries that can lead to this devastating fracture in women who may or may not have osteoporosis. These risk factors include frailty, muscle deconditioning, loss of coordination and balance, poor visual acuity and/or decreased depth perception, impaired hearing and associated dizziness, medications that compromise neuromuscular reflexes, and postural sway.

Patients with these risk factors should have a bone density test to confirm the diagnosis of osteoporosis. Patients who do not have osteoporosis should employ interventions to reduce fall risk (McClung et al., 2001).

2.25 What are the most useful interventions to prevent falls in older people living in their own homes?

A very useful intervention is a home exercise program to increase strength, flexibility, coordination, and posture. Such a program should include low-impact aerobics, resistance exercises (free weights, weight machines), balance (Tai Chi [Kessenich, 1998]), and flexibility (stretching). In addition, a comprehensive, progressive walking program, ambulatory aids when indicated, and instruction in proper body mechanics are helpful to reduce risk for falls and injuries.

2.26 What nonpharmacologic intervention is most effective to prevent hip fracture?

Hip protectors are undergarments that include a protective pad sewn into the hip region. The pads are designed to safely disperse the force of energy from a sideways fall away from the hip and into the soft tissue around the hip. Studies have shown that regular and consistent wearing of hip protectors can prevent many hip fractures (Lauritzen, Petersen, & Lund, 1993).

2.27 What are the general measures I can use to maintain healthy bones?

- Maintain a balanced diet with adequate intake of calcium and vitamin D. Calcium is an important nutrient for building bones in children and adolescents and for preventing bone loss in adults, especially in older men and women. Calcium is available through a person's diet (especially dairy products) or calcium supplements. Vitamin D is necessary for optimal calcium absorption from the intestine.
- Exercise: Weight-bearing exercise helps to build larger, stronger bones in children. In adults, regular exercise such as walking, dancing, lifting weights, and swimming can slow the rate of bone loss and can increase muscle strength. This decreases the likelihood of falls and fractures in older adults. Exercise sessions should last 30 minutes or more, three to four times per week.

- Avoid or stop smoking. Smoking increases the rate of bone loss, especially in postmenopausal women, and is associated with an increase in hip fracture risk compared to women who have never smoked. Although researchers have not clearly defined the relationship between smoking and osteoporosis, they know that women who smoke undergo menopause earlier and have lower circulating levels of estrogen than nonsmokers. The risk of fracture declines when smoking is stopped. The duration of smoking has more impact on fracture risk than the number of cigarettes smoked.
- Avoid excessive alcohol consumption. Excessive alcohol intake interrupts the function of cells that make new bone. Excessive alcohol intake (more than two drinks/day) also may lead to dietary insufficiencies, resulting in increased bone loss.
- Minimize use of medications that interfere with balance. These may include antidepressive drugs and some antihypertensive drugs. All women should talk with their healthcare providers about what options might be best for them.

References

Consensus Development Conference: Prophylaxis and treatment of osteoporosis. (1991). *Osteoporosis International, 1,* 114–126.

Cummings, S.R., Nevitt, M.C., Browner, W.S., Stone, K., Fox, K.M., & Ensrud, K.E. (1995). Risk factors for hip fracture in white women. *New England Journal of Medicine, 332,* 767–773.

Endocrine Nurses Society. (2002, October). *Diagnosis and treatment of postmenopausal osteoporosis: A guide for advanced health care professionals* [Continuing education offering from the Endocrine Nurses Society available from Interactive Network for Continuing Education]. Chevy Chase, MD: Author.

Ettinger, B., Black, D.M., Mitlak, B.H., Knickerbocker, R.K., Nickelsen, T., Genant, H.K., et al. (1999). Reduction of vertebral fracture risk in postmenopausal women with osteoporosis treated with raloxifene: Results from a 3-year randomized clinical trial. *JAMA, 282,* 637–645.

Harris, S.T., Watts, N.B., Genant, H.K., McKeever, C.D., Hingartner, T., Keller, M., et al. (1999). Effects of risedronate treatment on vertebral and nonvertebral fractures in women with postmenopausal osteoporosis: A randomized controlled trial. *JAMA, 282,* 1344–1352.

Hodgson, S.F., Watts, N.B., Bilezikian, J.P., Clarke, B.L., Gray, T.K., Harris, D.W., et al. (2001). American Association of Clinical Endocrinologists 2001 medical guidelines for clinical practice for the prevention and management of postmenopausal osteoporosis. *Endocrine Practice, 7,* 293–312.

Jergas, M., & Genant, H. (1993). Current methods and recent advances in the diagnosis of osteoporosis. *Arthritis and Rheumatism, 36,* 1649–1662.

Kessenich, C.R. (1998). Tai Chi as a method of fall prevention in the elderly. *Orthopaedic Nursing, 17*(4), 27–29.

Lauritzen, J.B., Petersen, M.M., & Lund, B. (1993). Effect of external hip protectors on hip fractures. *Lancet, 341,* 11–13.

Liberman, U.A., Weiss, S.R., Broll, J., Minne, H.W., Quan, H., Bell, N.H., et al. (1995). Effect of oral alendronate on bone mineral density and the incidence of fracture in postmenopausal women. *New England Journal of Medicine, 333,* 1437–1443.

McClung, M.R., Geusens, P., Miller, P.D., Zippel, H., Bensen, W.G., Roux, C., et al. (2001). Effect of risedronate on the risk of hip fracture in elderly women. *New England Journal of Medicine, 344,* 330–340.

Miller, P., Drezner, M., Delmas, J., Stakkestad, J., Hughes, C., Bonvoisin, B., et al. (2004). Monthly oral ibandronate in postmenopausal osteoporosis: 1-year results from MOBILE. *Journal of Bone and Mineral Research, 19*(Suppl. 1), S94.

National Institutes of Health Consensus Development Panel on Osteoporosis Prevention, Diagnosis, and Therapy. (2001). Osteoporosis prevention, diagnosis, and therapy. *JAMA, 285,* 785–795.

National Osteoporosis Foundation. (2003). *Physician's guide to prevention and treatment of osteoporosis.* Washington, DC: Author.

Neer, R.M., Arnaud, C.D., Zanchetta, J.R., Prince, R., Gaich, G.A., Reginster, J.Y., et al. (2001). Effect of parathyroid hormone (1-34) on fractures and bone mineral density in postmenopausal women with osteoporosis. *New England Journal of Medicine, 344,* 1434–1441.

Standing Committee on the Scientific Evaluation of Dietary Reference Intakes, Food and Nutrition Board, Institute of Medicine. (1997). *Dietary reference intakes for calcium, phosphorus, magnesium, vitamin D, and fluoride.* Washington, DC: National Academies Press.

WHO Study Group. (1994). *Assessment of fracture risk and its application to screening for postmenopausal osteoporosis.* Geneva, Switzerland: World Health Organization.

Resources

American Society for Bone and Mineral Research: www.asbmr.org
Foundation for Osteoporosis Research and Education: www.fore.org
International Osteoporosis Foundation: www.osteofound.org
International Society for Clinical Densitometry: www.iscd.org
National Institute for Arthritis and Musculoskeletal and Skin Diseases: www.niams.nih.gov
National Institutes of Health Osteoporosis and Related Bone Diseases National Resource Center: www.osteo.org
National Osteoporosis Foundation: www.nof.org
North American Menopause Society: www.menopause.org

Osteoporosis Patient Education Brochures

Endocrine Nurses Society: www.endo-nurses.org; a series of six brochures is available. Send your request via e-mail to ginny.wiatrowski@aurora.org
Osteoporosis Society of Canada: www.osteoporosis.ca; brochures and fact sheets are available free of charge by calling 800-463-6842.
U.S. Department of Health and Human Services. (2004). *The 2004 surgeon general's report on bone health and osteoporosis: What it means to you.* Rockville, MD: U.S. Department of Health and Human Services Office of the Surgeon General. Available online at www.surgeongeneral .gov/library/bonehealth/docs/OsteoBrochure1mar05.pdf

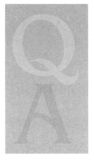

Chapter 3
Breast Health and Breast Cancer

Joanne Lester, MSN, RNC, CNP, AOCN®

Background

Q 3.1 No one in my family has breast cancer. Why do I need a mammogram?

In this case, it is fortunate that the woman does not have a family history of breast cancer. Depending on any other risk factors she may have, she most likely ranks with the average woman in the United States, with an 11%–12% chance of developing breast cancer in her lifetime. That figures out to 1 out of every 7–8 women. From what medical professionals know today, only 5%–10% of all breast cancers are hereditary, or genetically involved. Therefore, 90%–95% of breast cancers are not hereditary. In fact, most women who develop breast cancer have no risk factors at all except being a woman of increasing age (Jemal et al., 2006; Sifri, Gangadharappa, & Acheson, 2004).

Q 3.2 Do mammograms hurt? I do not want to get one if they do!

Although compression of the breast during a mammogram can be uncomfortable, this discomfort seldom lasts. Compression of the breast tissue is necessary to obtain an accurate assessment. Lester (2000) provided some suggestions to minimize tenderness experienced with a mammogram.
- Schedule a mammogram several days after the end of a menstrual period.
- Consider taking acetaminophen or ibuprofen (if compatible with other medication) the day prior to and day of a mammogram.
- Consider stopping hormone replacement therapy five to seven days prior to a mammogram; for some women, this reduces breast tenderness. (Note: Women should check with their physicians before changing medication patterns.)

• Decrease intake of coffee, tea, cola products, and chocolate because caffeine intake may contribute to breast tenderness.
• Inform the radiology technician of any tenderness so that additional interventions can be implemented to provide comfort.

Remember that mammography, with clinical exam and breast self-exam, is the primary tool in finding a breast cancer in its earliest stage. It is an important annual screening tool.

Q 3.3   Aren't annual mammograms harmful because of all the radiation exposure?

The radiation exposure from modern, low-dose mammography equipment is minimal. Each breast receives approximately one rad. The medical benefits of early detection far outweigh any potential risk.

Q 3.4   How can I check my breasts properly? I feel lumps all over and would be calling my healthcare provider every day because I would find something.

Monthly breast self-examinations remain an important tool in early detection of breast abnormalities and cancer. Women with fibrocystic breasts experience challenges with self-exam, as they may feel multiple lumps. Lester (2000) offers guidelines to help women to feel more comfortable.
• Examine breasts at the same time each month. Women who are still menstruating should perform breast self-examination after the period has ended, as their breasts soften and become less tender.
• Examine breasts with the flat section of three fingers, avoiding the use of only one fingertip. This will allow women to feel a larger area of tissue, realizing that each inch feels like the next inch. If women take one finger and individually feel each and every fibrocystic lump, their exam may be very confusing. If a woman notes a discrete lesion or thickening, she should see her physician.
• Ask a healthcare provider to demonstrate the technique of breast self-examination. Women should examine their breasts in both an upright position, such as in the shower, and while lying down in bed. Palpate available models in the office to discern lumps of concern versus fibrocystic changes of the breast.
• Remember that a patient's job is to identify any abnormality, not to decide whether it is something significant. Women should

report any new change in the breast to their physician and have it checked. If indeed the "lump" they feel is really okay, everyone will be relieved, including their physician.

3.5   I have fibrocystic breast disease. Does that increase my risk of breast cancer?

Fibrocystic breast disease is not really a disease but a normal condition of the breast that changes over a lifetime in relationship to hormone status (Bowen, Alfano, McGregor, & Andersen, 2004). Fibrocystic changes may confuse examination of the breast, making it more difficult to identify lumps. Mammograms can be more difficult to read because of dense white tissue on the films. For these reasons, a breast cancer may be more difficult to find at an early stage in women with significant amounts of fibrous breast tissue. A woman who has fibrocystic breast tissue is not at greater risk for developing breast cancer in her lifetime; it just may be more difficult to identify.

3.6   What about studies that say breast self-examination is not useful? Should I really do it?

Often the media misrepresent study results, or reported results may not be from a reputable study. Breast self-examination performed monthly by a woman in the privacy of her home continues to be an important part of breast health. Unfortunately, not all women undergo mammograms, and not all breast cancers show up on mammograms. Also, not all women go to their healthcare providers for an annual clinical breast exam. Therefore, women still need to perform breast self-examination. It is free, easy to do, and may save women's lives.

3.7   What can I do to get rid of fibrocystic tissue?

Again, in most women, fibrocystic breast tissue is a normal condition. Women who have functioning ovaries can have fibrocystic tissue related to their own hormonal status. Women who are postmenopausal without functioning ovaries often note a decrease in fibrous tissue over time. If a woman is taking any type of hormone therapy or using plant estrogens or soy products, decreasing use of these medications/supplements may decrease the amount of fibrocystic tissue (Horner & Lampe, 2000).

Q 3.8   I am 34 years old and have not had children yet. I feel my biological clock ticking because I know this is a risk factor for breast cancer. Are my concerns valid?

Various factors related to uninterrupted estrogen effects in women's bodies may slightly increase their incidence of breast cancer. Although these are important factors to consider in one's overall lifestyle, a woman does not *significantly* increase her risk of developing breast cancer related only to her age at childbirth. This is only one factor among many to be considered when determining a woman's risk (Bowen et al., 2004; Deane & Degner, 1998).

Q 3.9   My doctor says I can quit having mammograms once I turn 70 years old. Is this true?

The incidence of breast cancer in women increases with age; therefore, women should continue to have annual mammograms unless there is a health reason prohibiting this screening test (Jemal et al., 2006).

Q 3.10   I feel a lump but was told my mammogram is normal. What should I do?

A physician should clinically evaluate any breast lump with a breast examination. Unfortunately, mammograms only identify approximately 80% of breast cancers, meaning approximately 20% may not show up on mammograms. If a woman still has a concern about a lump after seeing her physician, she should consider a second opinion with a surgeon.

Prevention/Detection

Q 3.11   Hormone replacement therapy—should I take it or not?

As medical professionals continue to learn more about the benefits and risks of hormone replacement therapy, one thing is clear: Each woman needs individual assessment and counseling according to her individual risks of developing breast cancer, osteoporosis, heart disease, and menopausal symptoms. Certain risk factors, such as abnormal breast biopsies with atypical cells, lobular carcinoma *in situ*, or an actual diagnosis of ductal carcinoma *in situ* or invasive breast cancer preclude the use of hormone replacement therapy. Any woman with a strong family history of breast cancer in first-degree relatives (i.e., mother, daughter, sister) should limit the use of hormone replacement therapy and consider other alternatives for symptom relief (Bluming, 2004; Greenwald, 2005).

Q 3.12 What about taking any of the "natural" hormone products on the market?

Currently, no scientific data exist to support the benefits, risks, or efficacy of over-the-counter natural supplements or creams. No data exist to support that these products might be harmful, but then, no scientific data have shown that they are not harmful for high-risk women or breast cancer survivors. All of these products are based on plant estrogens that are manufactured, so are they really "natural" products? Until further scientific research supports their use and safety, it most likely is best to avoid using such products or to use them with caution. Women should discuss any supplements they are considering with a healthcare professional.

Q 3.13 My mother has breast cancer, and I feel doomed that I also will develop breast cancer. What can I do?

A number of factors determine a person's risk of developing breast cancer, including family history. Healthcare providers worry most about first-degree relatives (a mother, daughter, or sister, as well as a father, son, or brother) if those relatives developed breast cancer at an early age. In women, the age groups typically are split between premenopausal and postmenopausal. Women should talk with their healthcare providers regarding their specific risk factors. A number of interventions may be helpful if a strong family history exists.

• Women should consider seeing their healthcare providers twice a year for a clinical breast examination. They should obtain an annual mammogram and perform monthly breast self-examinations.

• Women need to discuss the use of hormone replacement therapy carefully with their healthcare providers; if women choose to use it, use of these drugs sould be limited (less than one to two years).

• Women may consider a consultation with a physician who focuses on breast health in high-risk women. Depending on a woman's personal risk factors, she may be eligible to take medications to help to lower her risk of developing breast cancer, such as antiestrogens, aromatase inhibitors, or possibly one of the other medications currently being studied for breast cancer prevention (Sifri et al., 2004).

Q 3.14   I have read that underwire bras and antiperspirants may increase the risk of developing breast cancer. Is this true?

No scientific data support a negative effect of either underwire bras or antiperspirants.

Q 3.15   My mother developed breast cancer at the age of 43. What screening recommendations should I follow?

For women with first-degree relatives with breast cancer, the rule of thumb is to start annual mammography screening 10 years prior to the age when the youngest first-degree relative developed breast cancer. In the case presented, this would be at age 33. In addition, twice-yearly clinical breast examinations by a physician and monthly self breast examinations would be recommended (Jemal et al., 2006; Sifri et al., 2004).

Q 3.16   I have a strong family history of breast cancer; what should I do? This includes my paternal grandmother (age 82), her sister (age 79), and my maternal first cousin (age 48).

In regard to family history of breast cancer, healthcare providers are most concerned about first-degree relatives. Second-degree relatives (grandmothers) are important but are less worrisome than first-degree relatives. In this case, the first cousin and great-aunt are less significant, being third-degree relatives (Sifri et al., 2004).

Q 3.17   I have a mother and sister with breast cancer and want to consider genetic testing. How do I accomplish that?

Ideally, a genetic team with appropriate assessment and counseling expertise should perform genetic testing. This team is most experienced in guiding patients in their decision making, insurability issues, lifestyle changes, and other important issues. The actual testing involves only a blood test. If possible, the team will draw blood from a family member with breast cancer before they perform a test on family members at risk. If the relative with breast cancer does not test positive for the genetic mutation, the genetic team may not perform the test on another relative who is seeking testing (Sifri et al., 2004).

Q 3.18   I have just been diagnosed with breast cancer. How can I find out about my mother's breast cancer to see if mine is genetically the same as hers?

If relatives with breast cancer are genetically positive, the positivity relates only to the fact that they developed the breast cancer and carry the gene mutation. The specific characteristics of the breast cancer are not necessarily genetically related and therefore cannot be predicted. Likewise, if a relative died of her disease, it does not genetically predict that other relatives also will die of their disease. The genetics relate only to the fact that the breast cancer occurred (Sifri et al., 2004).

3.19 **I tested positive for the breast cancer gene. I already have right breast cancer and have had a lumpectomy with radiation therapy. What should I do?**

The answer is not easy. Multiple factors must be considered. In relation to breast cancer, the woman in this situation could consider bilateral prophylactic mastectomies, although that may not be specifically recommended for her. The other area of potential concern is her ovaries, which are at risk related to her genetic positivity. It is difficult to identify ovarian cancer in an early stage; for that reason, preventive bilateral oophorectomy (removal of the ovaries) often is recommended as prevention in women who test gene positive. Unfortunately, this creates a surgical menopause (unless the patient is already menopausal). Healthcare professionals do not recommend hormone replacement therapy to relieve menopausal symptoms because of the women's breast cancer history, but other interventions are available. Once a woman is determined to be genetically positive, she should have discussions with her oncologist(s), gynecologist, and genetic team prior to making any decisions.

3.20 **What is the STAR trial?**

The STAR trial is a national study (National Cancer Institute [NCI], 2005) looking at the prevention of breast cancer in high-risk women. It stands for the **S**tudy of **T**amoxifen **A**nd **R**aloxifene in the prevention of breast cancer. The first prevention trial, P-1, studied tamoxifen versus placebo in high-risk women. Researchers stopped the study prematurely in 1998 because those women taking tamoxifen clearly showed a benefit, with an average of 49% improvement in the incidence of breast cancer. Therefore, all women in the study received the opportunity to take tamoxifen.

Simultaneously, another trial (the MORE trial—**M**ultiple **O**utcomes of **R**aloxifene **E**valuation) studying raloxifene for the prevention of osteoporosis was under way; women taking raloxifene showed a reduction in breast cancer incidence (NCI, 1999). The STAR study uses both of these drugs, tamoxifen and raloxifene, with the woman taking one or the other, in an attempt to determine which drug is better and which drug is better tolerated. Results of this study should soon be available.

3.21   What about other drugs to prevent breast cancer?

Researchers are studying another group of drugs, aromatase inhibitors, for their potential breast cancer prevention roles. Investigators also are studying aspirin, nonsteroidal anti-inflammatory drugs, cyclooxygenase (COX)-2 inhibitors, and various vitamins for possible prevention properties (Sifri et al., 2004). It is an exciting time as healthcare professionals critically look at breast cancer prevention. Women should talk with a healthcare provider or call NCI for more information.

3.22   I have read that ultrasound is better than mammography for detecting cancer in dense breast tissue. True?

Mammography remains the best diagnostic tool to radiographically detect breast changes and/or cancer. Ultrasound determines whether a lump that is felt or seen on mammogram is cystic (fluid filled) or solid. There is no evidence that ultrasound for the sole purpose of screening should be used instead of mammography. Therefore, healthcare professionals still recommend an annual mammogram with the possible addition of targeted ultrasound. In certain cases, they also may perform magnetic resonance imaging to better distinguish changes in breast tissue (Lester, 2000).

3.23   I have read that breast cancer does not hurt, but my breast cancer lump did.

Painful breast masses can be related to fibrocystic breast tissue/cysts. These account for many of the lumps that are found in women's breasts. A breast cancer can cause pain because it pulls at surrounding tissue. Often upon touching a breast cancer, a woman feels no pain. However, a healthcare provider should evaluate any lump that is found in a woman's breast, regardless of whether it hurts (Lester, 2000).

3.24   I need a breast biopsy. What are my options?

Today, a number of methods are available to biopsy lesions in the breast. For lesions that can be felt, three options are available: fine needle aspiration, core needle biopsy, or excisional biopsy. For lesions that only can be found on mammogram or ultrasound, options are ultrasound-guided core needle biopsy, needle localization excisional biopsy, or stereotactic biopsy (Deane & Degner, 1998). Which biopsy is performed depends on a number of factors. Women should ask their surgeons if a less-invasive type of biopsy is indicated in their situations.

Treatment

3.25   I have just been diagnosed with breast cancer and want to do everything possible. Can't they just remove both of my breasts?

It is a common response for women, upon hearing a breast cancer diagnosis, to want to do everything possible to increase their survival rate. Women generally are given options for the treatment of their breast cancer based on the suspected stage. Lumpectomy plus radiation therapy often is offered as a treatment, especially in the case of early-stage cancer. But, a mastectomy may be recommended because of the size of the tumor, location of the tumor within the breast, size of breast in relation to tumor size, or history of previous radiation therapy (Fisher et al., 2002).

If given the option between a lumpectomy and mastectomy, women should explore the pros and cons of each option in regard to their specific situations. Women need to give themselves "permission" to keep their breast(s), if that is what they desire. In turn, if women desire a mastectomy, it is their choice, as long as they realize they are not "doing more" for their cancer treatment. Although a mastectomy may feel like a more aggressive treatment, scientifically, a lumpectomy plus radiation therapy is equal to a mastectomy (Fisher et al., 2002).

When diagnosed with breast cancer, it is important to consider both the local treatment (the breast) and the systemic treatment (the whole body). From the very beginning, an invasive breast cancer is thought of as a systemic disease. Local treatment consists of lumpectomy with radiation therapy or mastectomy with or without radiation therapy. Systemic treatment consists of chemotherapy and/or hormonal therapy.

A number of variables exist in regard to breast-conserving surgery (lumpectomy) versus mastectomy (Cianfrocca & Goldstein, 2004). If a woman is eligible for a lumpectomy and radiation, a mastectomy will not improve her chance of cure. If cells have escaped into the lymph or circulatory systems, taking more breast tissue will not accomplish anything systemically. Studies have proved that a lumpectomy with radiation therapy equals a mastectomy in regard to local treatment unless reasons prevail for why more tissue must be removed (Fisher et al., 2002).

Some women discuss removing both of their breasts—one mastectomy to treat the breast cancer and one mastectomy as prevention. Again, removing more tissue, especially a noncancerous breast, will not add any benefit to the overall survival. Often healthcare professionals recommend that women have their definitive surgery with determination of the stage of their breast cancer before making a decision for bilateral mastectomies. For example, if a woman has her definitive breast cancer surgery, and it is determined to be a high stage based on tumor size and lymph node status, then clinicians may place urgency on systemic treatment, not more aggressive surgery. Patients should consider many factors when a breast cancer diagnosis occurs, and facts, not fear, should guide decisions. Patients should consider a second opinion if they are unsure of what direction to take (Hiotis, Ye, Sposto, & Skinner, 2005).

Q 3.26   I have been diagnosed with breast cancer and must have a mastectomy. Why can't I keep my nipple?

This is a vital structure of the breast and most often receives treatment either surgically with removal or with radiation therapy. If surgeons perform a mastectomy, they routinely remove all of the breast tissue, surrounding skin, and nipple. If they perform reconstruction, they can fashion an artificial nipple that often looks very normal.

Q 3.27   I do not want to have my lymph nodes removed. Are there any other options?

The axillary lymph nodes routinely undergo surgical assessment with a breast cancer diagnosis. This is important in determining the stage of a patient's disease. Many times with a newly diagnosed breast cancer, physicians can perform a procedure called sentinel lymph node biopsy. The sentinel node is the first node that drains the breast cancer. If healthcare professionals can accurately identify the sentinel node, then they can determine the stage of the breast cancer without removing all of the axillary lymph nodes.

This procedure involves injecting the breast with a radioactive substance and blue dye the day of surgery. During surgery, physicians identify the sentinel lymph node in the axilla and remove and test it for cancer cells. If they see no cancer cells, they often leave the remaining nodes in the axilla. However, if they find cancer cells in the sentinel lymph node, surgeons often proceed with a routine axillary node dissection (Cianfrocca & Goldstein, 2004).

Q 3.28   My sentinel lymph node was normal at the time of surgery but positive when the final pathologic results came back. Do I need to have my remaining lymph nodes removed?

This is a difficult question that does not have an exact answer. The decision to perform, or not perform, a subsequent axillary node dissection depends upon a number of variables specific to each person and her breast cancer. Several studies are under way to determine whether a subsequent axillary node dissection is necessary for all women (Cianfrocca & Goldstein, 2004).

Q 3.29   My lymph nodes were removed. What are my chances of developing lymphedema?

When physicians surgically remove axillary lymph nodes, women, as well as healthcare professionals, must take precautions to prevent permanent swelling in the affected arm (lymphedema). If these precautions are taken, most women do not experience swelling or infections in the arm. Less than one-third of all women will develop significant lymphedema following axillary node dissection, and the vast majority of women do not develop permanent problems. If swelling or infection appears, it is important to intervene quickly to prevent permanent damage and side effects.

Q 3.30   I have breast cancer and had my lymph nodes removed more than five years ago. I have been told to avoid blood pressure readings and blood draws in that arm. When I go to my doctor's office, they say it is okay to use that arm. What is the right answer?

Once the axillary lymph nodes are surgically removed, the arm on that side of the body is at risk for developing lymphedema and infection. A number of precautions exist, including avoidance of blood pressures, blood draws, needle sticks, injections, lying on that arm, cuts and bug bites, and gardening without gloves. This is a lifetime risk; therefore, patients should practice the precautions for a lifetime.

Q 3.31   **My axillary lymph nodes have been removed on both sides. Where should I have blood drawn and my blood pressure taken?**

When a woman has bilateral axillary node dissections (lymph nodes removed from both armpits), it can present a problem. Ideally, healthcare professionals should take blood pressures in the thigh, and patients should purchase a special cuff to take to physician visits. Nurses should obtain blood draws from the foot, if possible, or from the "oldest" arm with a very light tourniquet. If surgery or hospitalization is necessary, nurses often will place the IV in a vein in the neck to avoid using the arms. The patient should receive injections in the hip (intramuscular) or abdominal/thigh tissue (subcutaneous). In an emergency, regard for one's life supersedes the possible risk of lymphedema.

Q 3.32   **Should I wear a compression sleeve to prevent lymphedema when taking an airline flight?**

No scientific data exist to support that airline flights induce lymphedema, although a number of factors may be involved. Women should avoid carrying heavy suitcases with their affected arm, pulling suitcases on wheels through the airport, and lifting heavy items into overhead bins. If traveling on a long flight, they must frequently move their arm to avoid swelling related to immobility. They should consider taking a small rubber ball to squeeze and raise their arm in the air several times an hour. If their arm is prone to swelling and they already have experienced problems with lymphedema, then it would be advisable for them to wear a compression sleeve while in flight.

Q 3.33   **My tumor was estrogen positive, but I have never taken estrogen. How can that be?**

Breast cancer cells undergo testing for a variety of factors, including estrogen and progesterone receptors. Presence of these receptors is a characteristic of the cancer and cannot show whether women are pre- or postmenopausal or whether they were taking hormones. Many premenopausal women have estrogen-receptor/progesterone-receptor–negative tumors, whereas most postmenopausal women have receptor-positive tumors.

It is most desirable to be estrogen- and progesterone-receptor positive because these tumors tend to behave in a better manner. This status also enables a woman to use hormonal agents, such as antiestrogens and/or aromatase inhibitors, to systemically treat her breast cancer.

3.34   There are so many antiestrogen drugs. Which one(s) should I take?

Systemic therapy for breast cancer may include the use of hormonal agents. Typically, a woman must be estrogen positive and/or progesterone positive to take these medications. These drugs are designed to prevent absorption of estrogen by certain receptors on the breast cancer cell or to temporarily or permanently disrupt the estrogen pathway to the cancer cell. Results of various studies using these drugs indicate that combining or sequencing these drugs over years may be beneficial.

At the current time, confusion can occur over which drug(s) to take and in which order. The only definite answer is that premenopausal women can take only antiestrogens (unless menopause is induced), whereas postmenopausal women potentially can take antiestrogens and/or aromatase inhibitors. The most exciting thing about this confusion is that so many options are available for women with breast cancer. As researchers continue to learn more through clinical trial results, the answers will become clearer (Takusugi et al., 2005).

3.35   If I have breast reconstruction, will it decrease the physician's ability to detect a recurrence of my cancer?

Most breast cancers recur systemically, meaning elsewhere in the body. A small percent chance exists of a breast cancer recurring on the chest wall. Except for certain circumstances, having reconstruction at the time of the mastectomy or later on will not hinder follow-up or the detection of recurrence at the mastectomy site.

3.36   Why have I been diagnosed with breast cancer? I never smoked or drank to excess. I have always exercised and taken care of myself. How could this have happened?

Unfortunately, it is not evident why women develop breast cancer. In this case, nothing the woman has done has made this breast cancer happen. Thankfully, she has taken very good care of herself, is healthy, and her body is in good shape. Therefore, she should be able to do whatever it takes to maximize her outcome with this diagnosis.

Side Effects

3.37   **I always said I would never take chemotherapy, but now that I've been diagnosed with breast cancer, I am considering it. I only know horror stories about the side effects. Will I be able to tolerate chemotherapy?**

It is easy for people to make a "decision" against taking chemotherapy when there is no actual threat to their health. However, when a cancer diagnosis is made, they are faced with reality. Patients with cancer must consider all treatment options for the best chance of controlling the disease. Healthcare professionals routinely use chemotherapy after a newly diagnosed breast cancer to treat the whole body for microscopic metastasis. Over the years, the mortality rates for breast cancer have started to decline, in part, because of the use of chemotherapy. Most women with breast cancer are healthy, which makes tolerating chemotherapy a little easier. Many of the "horror" stories related to chemotherapy involve people who are very ill with their cancer who also suffer the debilitating side effects of chemotherapy and succumb to their disease. Although breast cancer chemotherapy has its side effects, patients tolerate it fairly well overall. More importantly, for many women, it can make an impact on their disease process, with the hope of eliminating metastatic disease in the future.

3.38   **I have heard that although I need radiation therapy to my breast, a new procedure is available that eliminates radiating the whole breast. Is this true?**

Traditionally, women who have a lumpectomy must follow with whole breast radiation therapy that consists of daily treatments, Monday through Friday, for six to seven weeks. Although this radiation typically is very well tolerated, it radiates the entire breast and underlying structures. Researchers are conducting studies with localized radiation therapy to the origin of the tumor as opposed to radiation therapy to the whole breast. This can be accomplished in a number of ways but typically limits the course of radiation to less than one week. Clinical trials are in process to evaluate the final decisions regarding this exciting, time-limited approach.

3.39   Will I lose my hair with radiation therapy?

Radiation works where it is pointed, so the side effects are related to the target area. Therefore, radiation therapy only causes hair loss when the head or brain is radiated. Radiation therapy to the breast can cause skin changes such as sunburning, tenderness, and thickening. It also can cause fatigue, which may be related, in part, to the daily trips for the six to seven weeks of treatment. Overall, patients tolerate breast radiation therapy fairly well.

3.40   Will I lose my hair during chemotherapy? Will it come back?

Most breast cancer chemotherapy regimens include drugs that induce complete hair loss. This loss typically occurs two weeks after initiation of the regimen if certain drugs, such as anthracyclines, are used. Sometimes the hair loss is gradual, and other times it is a dramatic loss over a couple of days. With hair loss related to breast cancer chemotherapy, hair growth always returns. Resources for attractive wigs, hats, and hair coverings are available in most communities. If such products are not readily available, the American Cancer Society (ACS) has a large selection of products that can be purchased online or by mail. Some local chapters of ACS provide wigs and hair coverings free of charge.

Post-Treatment Issues

3.41   Can you scan my body to make sure I do not have disease anywhere else? What about blood tests?

When a woman is newly diagnosed with breast cancer, the body scans that used to be routinely performed often are no longer done. If a woman has significant disease such as inflammatory or locally advanced cancer, or if after surgery multiple lymph node involvement is found, bone scans and computed tomography scans often are performed at that time. Otherwise, these are not routinely performed unless a woman exhibits symptoms to warrant such a test. These guidelines are developed by a national committee guiding cancer care, the National Comprehensive Cancer Network (NCCN, 2005). To view the NCCN patient or physician guidelines, please visit www.nccn.org. One would think that, technologically, instruments are available that can measure microscopic disease elsewhere in the body, but such tests do not exist. Most often, if a patient with breast cancer has metastatic disease, she will exhibit symptoms that guide her physician to detect the abnormality with appropriate imaging studies.

Currently, no reliable blood tests exist that accurately diagnose breast cancer or early recurrence. Tumor markers sensitive to breast cancer, such as CEA and CA 15-3 (or CA 27-29), sometimes are used to monitor metastatic disease and its progress, but they are not routinely measured otherwise (Cianfrocca & Goldstein, 2004).

3.42   How can I control my hot flashes if I cannot take hormone replacement therapy?

Breast cancer survivors who need to avoid the use of estrogen can implement a number of interventions to minimize or eliminate hot flashes related to menopause. Simple ideas such as wearing light layers of cotton clothing, maintaining cooler room temperatures, and drinking ice water work for many women. Eliminating or reducing caffeine and alcohol intake often makes an impact. Vitamin E, if recommended by a physician, often is helpful. Also, a number of other medications that are used for other reasons may benefit women with uncontrollable hot flashes and can be prescribed by physicians. This includes drugs such as certain antidepressants, hypotensive agents, antispasmodics, or anticonvulsants (Zibecchi, Greendale, & Ganz, 2003). Women should communicate with their healthcare providers to identify specific interventions to aid them.

3.43   Is there any help for my vaginal dryness?

Again, breast cancer survivors and high-risk women typically avoid the use of estrogen for vaginal dryness. A number of effective over-the-counter water-soluble lubricants are available. These products evaporate very quickly, so sufficient amounts should be used to provide adequate lubrication. It is recommended, if important to a woman, to engage in sexual activity on a regular basis, as a woman's own natural lubrication provides much internal moisture.

Topical hormone creams often are not recommended because of potential systemic absorption, although small amounts used infrequently may be acceptable. Products that are estradiol based but have very little systemic absorption are available through physicians. These are thought to be safe for three to six months of use. Further research needs to be performed to verify the safety and efficacy of these products in breast cancer survivors.

Q 3.44   What can I do to prevent osteoporosis if I cannot take hormone replacement therapy?

It is important to monitor a woman's bone density, especially if her menopause was induced by chemotherapy. Studies have shown that these women have an increased risk of developing osteoporosis at an earlier age than their counterparts. Routine bone dual x-ray absorptiometry scans should be performed, as well as encouraging supplemental calcium intake and routine weight-bearing exercise. If bone loss occurs, a number of interventions are safe for breast cancer survivors that can improve and restore density. Hormone replacement therapy is not the current approach for the prevention of osteoporosis in any woman, regardless of whether she has breast cancer.

It is very important to monitor bone density in women who are taking hormonal agents that interrupt the estrogen pathway. These include aromatase inhibitors, as these drugs have been shown to potentially decrease bone density in postmenopausal women. Antiestrogens, on the other hand, often can improve bone density for women (Zibecchi et al., 2003).

Q 3.45   Can I safely get pregnant after a breast cancer diagnosis?

The answer is unknown, but no scientific data support that pregnancy after a breast cancer diagnosis is harmful. Often, chemotherapy induces menopause even in younger women. In this case, future attempts at pregnancy are unsuccessful. It is recommended that a woman wait a period of time after diagnosis and the completion of treatments to ensure a safe and healthy pregnancy for herself and the baby. Science cannot say exactly what that time period is, but oncologists tend to recommend at least two years following the end of treatment(s) and possibly longer. It is important that women not get pregnant while on medications to treat breast cancer, such as chemotherapy or antiestrogens, as the effects on the fetus are unknown.

Q 3.46   Will I resume my menstrual periods after chemotherapy is over?

No one ever knows the answer to that question until it happens. Chemotherapy can induce a temporary or permanent chemical menopause. It is not unusual for women to go 12–18 months, or even longer, without a cycle and then restart. Therefore, birth control measures should be practiced. Overall, if a woman does not cycle for a full year after completion of her chemotherapy, permanent menopause is considered to have occurred.

Q 3.47   Can't I have a blood test to find out if I am in menopause?

Several blood tests exist that can attempt to determine menopausal status, although no sure way is available. In all women experiencing "the change of life," the transition to a postmenopausal status is confounded by fluctuating hormone levels. This makes blood tests difficult to evaluate, as women can experience hormonal surges and/or deficits at various points in this transition. Breast cancer survivors complicate this evaluation even further with the potential hormonal side effects related to chemotherapy and hormonal agents, such as antiestrogens and/or aromatase inhibitors. Therefore, a woman should protect herself from pregnancy until a full year has passed without a menstrual cycle or spotting. Then, with the help of her gynecologist and oncologist(s), a possible determination can be made. Even with a full year without menstrual cycles, women who are taking hormonal agents could resume their cycles. It can be a very frustrating time for women, but it eventually will end with the inevitable confirmation of a postmenopausal status.

Q 3.48   I have been told I will be prescribed antiestrogen therapy. What are the negative side effects?

Antiestrogen drugs are some of the most researched drugs in the United States, having been studied in more than 10 million women for more than the past 25 years. Antiestrogens are excellent drugs for the control of breast cancer and the prevention of metastatic disease. However, they carry some potentially negative side effects.
- Can increase menopausal symptoms such as hot flashes and vaginal dryness
- Can cause a less than 1% increased risk of developing blood clots; this is the same risk as when taking birth control pills, fertility drugs, or hormone replacement therapy.
- Can cause a less than 1% increased risk of developing uterine/endometrial cancer, which most often is diagnosed through vaginal spotting or bleeding. Although the literature may report this information as "the risk of uterine cancer is increased 3–4 more times if taking antiestrogen drugs," this translates to 3–4 women

per 1,000 women, which still calculates to less than 1% overall. Remember, statistics can be very confusing unless a person knows the context in which they are described.

Overall, antiestrogen drugs play a very important role and are excellent drugs that should not be feared. Other hormonal agents, such as aromatase inhibitors, are available and may be recommended for postmenopausal breast cancer survivors. However, side effects also may be experienced with these drugs (Takusugi et al., 2005).

3.49   I do not want to take antiestrogen drugs because I have heard they make you gain weight. Is this true?

Studies with antiestrogens and placebos clearly uphold that women taking the placebo gained more weight than women on the antiestrogens. Antiestrogens may increase one's appetite, so women should be careful not to increase their dietary caloric intake. If women take antiestrogens with the intent that they will not gain weight, and if they watch their calories and exercise regularly, they often can successfully control their weight.

3.50   What diet should I eat to avoid breast cancer or any recurrence of disease?

No specific dietary practices have been scientifically proven to prevent or treat breast cancer, although continued study in regard to low dietary fat intake shows promise. Women should eat a low-fat, healthy diet that includes multiple servings of fruits and vegetables. Concerns exist surrounding a high-fat intake or being overweight and their potential contributions to the occurrence and/or recurrence of breast cancer, as fat cells store estrogen. Overall, avoiding high-fat diets and maintaining a recommended weight throughout one's life is a sensible approach. Studies continue to determine the best preventive dietary habits (Greenwald, 2005). Until further research is completed, women should enjoy foods in moderation while controlling their weight and eating healthy, balanced meals.

3.51   Japanese women have a much lower incidence of breast cancer. Is this because of their high intake of dietary soy? Some of the health magazines say so.

Although Japanese women statistically have a lower incidence of breast cancer, it is unknown whether a single variable such as dietary soy is responsible. A number of differences exist between Japan and the United States that make it difficult to clearly link breast cancer prevention only to dietary soy intake. Until further studies are completed to determine the relationship between dietary soy and breast cancer, women at high risk for breast cancer and breast cancer survivors should avoid eating large amounts of dietary soy.

References

Bluming, A.Z. (2004). Hormone replacement therapy: The debate should continue. *Geriatrics, 59*(11), 35–37.

Bowen, D.J., Alfano, C.M., McGregor, B.A., & Andersen, M.R. (2004). The relationship between perceived risk, affect, and health behaviors. *Cancer Detection and Prevention, 28,* 409–417.

Cianfrocca, M., & Goldstein, L.J. (2004). Prognostic and predictive factors in early-stage breast cancer. *Oncologist, 9,* 606–616.

Deane, K.A., & Degner, L.F. (1998). Information needs, uncertainty and anxiety in women who had a breast biopsy with benign outcome. *Cancer Nursing, 21,* 117–126.

Fisher, B., Anderson, S., Bryant, J., Margolese, R.G., Deutsch, M., Fisher, E.R., et al. (2002). Twenty-year follow-up of a randomized trial comparing total mastectomy, lumpectomy, and lumpectomy plus irradiation for the treatment of invasive breast cancer. *New England Journal of Medicine, 347,* 1233–1241.

Greenwald, P. (2005). Lifestyle and medical approaches to cancer prevention. *Recent Results in Cancer Research, 166,* 1–15.

Hiotis, K., Ye, W., Sposto, R., & Skinner, K.A. (2005). Predictors of breast conservation therapy: Size is not all that matters. *Cancer, 103,* 892–899.

Horner, N.K., & Lampe, J.W. (2000). Potential mechanisms of diet therapy for fibrocystic breast conditions show inadequate evidence of effectiveness. *Journal of the American Dietetic Association, 100,* 1368–1380.

Jemal, A., Siegel, R., Ward, E., Murray, T., Xu, J., Smigal, C., et al. (2006). Cancer statistics, 2006. *CA: A Cancer Journal for Clinicians, 56,* 106–130.

Lester, J. (2000). Breast tenderness/nipple discharge/swelling/lumps. In D. Camp-Sorrell & R.A. Hawkins (Eds.), *Clinical manual for the oncology advanced practice nurse* (pp. 921–925). Pittsburgh, PA: Oncology Nursing Society.

National Cancer Institute. (1999, June). *Publication of the MORE trial results supports study of tamoxifen and raloxifene (STAR).* Retrieved September 12, 2005, from http://www.cancer. gov/newscenter/more

National Cancer Institute. (2005, September). *Study of tamoxifen and raloxifene (STAR) trial.* Retrieved September 12, 2005, from http://www.cancer.gov/clinicaltrials/digestpage/STAR

National Comprehensive Cancer Network. (2005, August). *Breast cancer treatment guidelines for patients—version VII.* Jenkintown, PA: Author. Retrieved February 8, 2006, from http://www. nccn.org/patients/patient_gls/_english/_breast/contents.asp

Sifri, R., Gangadharappa, S., & Acheson, L. (2004). Identifying and testing for hereditary susceptibility to common cancers. *CA: A Cancer Journal for Clinicians, 54,* 309–326.

Takusugi, M., Iwamoto, E., Akashi-Tanaka, S., Kinoshita, T., Fukutomi, T., & Kubouchi, K. (2005). General aspects and specific issues of informed consent on breast cancer treatments. *Breast Cancer, 12,* 39–44.

Zibecchi, L., Greendale, G., & Ganz, P. (2003). Comprehensive menopausal assessment: An approach to managing vasomotor and urogenital symptoms in breast cancer survivors. *Oncology Nursing Forum, 30,* 393–407.

Resources

American Cancer Society: www.cancer.org
National Cancer Institute: www.cancer.gov
National Comprehensive Cancer Network: www.nccn.org
Oncology Nursing Society: www.ons.org

Chapter 4

Gynecologic Cancers

Marcella Williams, MS, RN, AOCN®

Background

Gynecologic cancers are malignancies that affect the female organs of reproduction and the genitalia. Collectively, these cancers comprise approximately 13% of cancers in women (Jemal et al., 2006; Martin, 2004). Screening has been particularly beneficial in reducing mortality in cervical cancer. However, an effective screening tool for other gynecologic cancers remains elusive and cost prohibitive. General risk factors include age, family history, and endogenous or exogenous hormonal factors. These may include age at onset of menstruation, age at or lack of pregnancy, and age at menopause, as well as exposure to hormonal manipulation, including birth control methods and hormonal treatment for gynecologic conditions or symptoms of menopause. Interestingly, hormonal manipulation that may protect a woman from one type of cancer may simultaneously increase her risk for another. Therefore, women must be active and knowledgeable participants in decisions regarding hormonal therapy, and practitioners must be diligent in balancing each individual's risks and benefits.

4.1 **Are the "gynecologic cancers" all the same kind of cancer, just in different organs?**

No. Although the cervix and uterus are, in essence, a continuous organ, the presenting symptoms, diagnostic tests, and treatments for these two cancers are different. Ovarian cancer alone has multiple different cell types. Presentation, diagnosis, and treatment also vary.

4.2 **I am adopted. How can I evaluate my risk for developing cancer without knowledge of my birth parents' medical history?**

As with breast cancer, family history is an important component of a woman's risk for many of the gynecologic cancers. In the absence of this information, women should carefully consider the risks and benefits of any hormonal treatment and communicate clearly with their primary healthcare team if such decisions are necessary. Family history is not the only risk factor involved with gynecologic cancers. Women should be knowledgeable about cancer prevention and early detection. It is important that women heighten their awareness of warning signs and symptoms and seek routine screening appropriate for gynecologic malignancies.

4.3   How does the age of menarche and menopause affect a woman's risk for cancer?

Late menopause (after age 55), infertility, and nulliparity are associated with an increased risk for both ovarian and uterine cancers, whereas early menarche (before age 12) is associated with an increased risk for ovarian cancer.

4.4   Are there any connections between cancer and birth control methods?

Healthcare professionals suspect that uterine and ovarian cancers are hormonally related, in part, because of the association between these cancers and major hormonal experiences in a woman's lifetime. Specific research related to birth control pills and an increased risk of cancer has shown a decreased risk of both ovarian and uterine cancers but a slightly increased risk of breast cancer (Spinelli, Whitaker, & Birk, 2003). An increase in cervical cancer incidence among women using birth control pills may be related to the decreased likelihood of use of concurrent barrier contraception, such as condoms. Clinical trials investigating breast cancer prevention through the use of antiestrogen agents also revealed a slightly increased risk for uterine cancer.

4.5   How does hormone replacement therapy affect the risk of cancer development?

Recent research studies following postmenopausal women who use estrogen-only therapy to control menopausal symptoms revealed a significantly increased risk for the development of ovarian cancer. Subsequently, lower-dose estrogen in combination with progesterone therapy is now recommended, if hormone replacement therapy is used at all. Combination therapy does not seem to pose a significant risk; however, this relatively new treatment has not had large-scale long-term follow-up to confirm results (Spinelli et al., 2003).

Q __4.6__ **Do women with gynecologic cancer have to get chemotherapy, or can the cancer just be cut out?**

Treatment decisions for gynecologic cancers are dependent upon the type and stage of the disease. Surgery remains a mainstay for all of the solid tumors, but surgery is used in combination with radiation and chemotherapy for cancer that has spread beyond a small, confined area. Early detection for cervical cancer via screening Pap smears has greatly reduced the incidence of metastatic disease. Nevertheless, in the presence of invasive tumor growth or metastasis to lymph nodes, chemotherapy and radiation have a useful role in disease management. Unfortunately, the lack of good screening techniques for uterine and ovarian cancers means these cancers often are discovered after the disease is advanced. Therefore, surgery often will play an initial role in treatment, but chemotherapy and radiation usually are part of the postsurgical treatment plan.

Cervical Cancer

Cervical cancer was the number-one cancer killer of women in the past. The development and widespread use of the Pap smear as an effective screening tool has allowed early detection and treatment of this cancer, resulting in dramatically improved survival rates. Cervical cancer rates remain high in developing countries. In the United States, nearly 50% of women diagnosed with cervical cancer have never had a Pap smear (Martin, 2004). Additionally, incidence rates are higher in the uninsured, older adult, and minority populations with limited access to or use of Pap smear screening.

Q __4.7__ **Is it really important to have a Pap smear every year?**

The American Cancer Society revised its screening recommendation in 2002 and now suggests that screening begin approximately three years after the onset of vaginal intercourse and no later than age 21. Screening should continue annually with conventional testing or every two years using a more specific liquid-based cytology. If, at the age of 30, women have had three consecutive normal cytology results, they may be screened every two to three years, provided no other risk factors are present. For example, women who are HIV positive, were exposed to diethylstilbestrol in utero, or are immunocompromised because of steroidal treatment, chemotherapy, or organ transplantation therapy should continue annual screening. Screening can be discontinued after the age of 70 with three or more consecutive negative cytology tests and no positive tests in the past decade (Martin, 2004).

 4.8   **Is there any link between sexually transmitted diseases and cancer development?**

Yes and no. Cervical cancer essentially is considered a sexually transmitted disease because of the direct causative link between infection with human papilloma virus (HPV) and the development of cervical cancer. DNA of the HPV virus has been found in 93%–100% of cervical squamous cell carcinomas (Martin, 2004). This DNA is transmitted during sexual activity. HPV seems to be a necessary precursor to the development of cervical cancer but is not an isolated precursor to the disease. In fact, the majority of women infected with HPV will not develop cervical cancer. Simultaneously, no causal relationship between other sexually transmitted diseases and the development of cervical cancer has been clearly demonstrated. In June 2006, the U.S. Food and Drug Administration (FDA) approved Gardasil® (Merck, Whitehouse Station, NJ), a vaccine that prevents cervical cancer, precancerous lesions, and genital warts caused by HPV types 6, 11, 16, and 18.

4.9   **Do tampons increase your risk for cervical cancer?**

No evidence exists that shows tampon use is related to cervical cancer.

4.10   **I have had a dilatation and curettage (D&C) in the past. Will that increase my risk for cervical cancer?**

Minor surgical procedures will not alter the cellular structure of cervical tissue. Malignancy develops on a cellular level and is correlated with factors that alter cellular function or genetic makeup. Examples include smoking and exposure to HPV.

4.11   **I have had an abnormal Pap smear in the past that was treated with cryosurgery. Does that put me at increased risk for cervical cancer? What are the signs and symptoms I should watch for?**

Yes. If a woman has been diagnosed with a confined cancerous or precancerous lesion in the past, close follow-up is a very important part of her care. Thin, watery, blood-tinged vaginal drainage may be noted intermittently as an early sign of cervical cancer. Vaginal bleeding after sexual intercourse or douching is another sign. The vaginal bleeding usually increases as the cancer grows. Pain is considered a late sign of cervical cancer and may be present in the flank or leg.

4.12   What is a false-positive test result?

All tests, including the Pap smear, have some degree of false results, reflected by the sensitivity and specificity of the particular test. A false-positive test is an abnormal cytology in the absence of true disease. The liquid-based Pap is considered equivalent to the conventional Pap smear and has been approved by the FDA. Most studies have shown improved sensitivity. HPV-DNA testing with cytology also is commercially available, but the optimal use of this testing is not entirely clear because of the high cost of the equipment and testing resources needed. At this point, the technology remains promising and most likely will be used for women at high risk (Program for Appropriate Technology in Health, 2001).

4.13   What treatment options exist for cervical cancer?

Treatment decisions are varied based on the clinical stage of the disease at diagnosis, tumor bulk, and spread patterns. Generally, surgical treatment for very early cancer may involve colposcopic biopsy, traditional cone biopsy, laser, cryosurgery, or electrosurgical techniques. Microscopically invasive cancer may be treated with conization, hysterectomy, or intracavitary radiation. Bilateral lymph node dissection, chemotherapy, and pelvic external beam radiation are added in the presence of more locally advanced cancer. Cisplatin-based chemotherapy given concurrently with radiation therapy currently is considered standard treatment for advanced cervical cancer (Martin, 2004).

4.14   My friend was diagnosed with cervical cancer after she got pregnant. What can she do?

Preinvasive lesions usually are not treated during pregnancy, but expert colposcopy is necessary to rule out the presence of invasive cancer. Treatment for invasive tumors depends on the stage of the cancer and gestational age of the fetus at diagnosis. Traditionally, immediate treatment for cervical cancer is suggested in early pregnancy, and treatment is postponed if the cancer is found near the time of fetal maturity. Some case studies have suggested that delaying treatment to allow viability of the pregnancy may be a reasonable option for early-stage cervical cancer.

Uterine Cancer

Uterine cancer is the most common of the gynecologic malignancies and occurs primarily in postmenopausal women. Endometrial cancer (adenocarcinoma) arises from the lining of the uterus, the endometrium, and is the most prevalent type of uterine cancer. Other cell types, including papillary serous, squamous cell, clear cell, and uterine sarcoma, are more rare. The use of birth control pills for at least one year has been shown to reduce the risk of endometrial cancer. In fact, the benefit of using birth control pills persists for 15 years after use has been discontinued. Hysterectomy is the primary surgical treatment for uterine cancer. Treatment with hormonal therapy may prolong time to disease recurrence, and advanced disease is treated with chemotherapy. Radiation therapy may be used in nonsurgical patients or to palliate symptoms of advanced disease (Meunier, 2005).

4.15   Is it true that you are at increased risk for uterine cancer if you are childless or have children late in life?

Yes. Risk factors for uterine cancer include age older than 50, Caucasian race, obesity, nulliparity, infertility, dysfunctional uterine bleeding during menopause, early menarche, late menopause, diabetes, hypertension, estrogen-only therapy, antiestrogen therapy use, polycystic ovarian syndrome, and hyperplasia of the endometrium (Martin, 2004).

4.16   What are the warning signs of uterine cancer?

Symptoms of uterine cancer include unusual vaginal bleeding or discharge, painful or difficult urination, painful intercourse, or general pelvic pain.

4.17   My mother has "fibroids." What does this mean? Does it put me at risk for cancer?

Fibroids are nonmalignant tumors that develop in the uterine muscle. They frequently are found in women in their 40s and can cause irregular bleeding, pain, frequent urination, and vaginal discharge. A personal or family history of fibroids is not considered a risk factor for endometrial cancer or any other type of malignancy. However, medical monitoring of this condition is appropriate.

Q 4.18   How is uterine cancer diagnosed?

Annual pelvic exams, particularly for women older than age 40, are an important part of detecting uterine cancer. Diagnosis is made with aspiration curettage or endometrial biopsy, and a fractional D&C is performed to confirm diagnosis. Imaging studies such as computed tomography scan, magnetic resonance imaging, or ultrasound may be used to aid in the detection of uterine cancer.

Q 4.19   I am undergoing treatment for endometriosis. How will this affect my risk of having cancer in the future?

Endometriosis is a common, benign condition occuring in women in their 30s and 40s that involves overgrowth of endometrial tissue outside of the uterus. Endometriosis is treated with antiestrogen hormonal therapy. No reported risk has been associated with treatment of endometriosis and uterine cancer development.

Ovarian Cancer

Ovarian cancer is the fifth leading cause of death in women of all ages. This cancer has been called "the silent killer" for its vague presenting symptoms that often lead to diagnosis well after metastasis has occured. Advocacy groups stress the importance of clinically investigating abdominal symptoms, such as widening girth, feelings of being bloated, and weight gain.

Q 4.20   I have had a hysterectomy. Why do I still need pelvic exams?

Pelvic examination is used for detection of ovarian cancer and therefore is recommended. A Pap smear still will be performed if the cervix was left intact. This varies depending on the surgical procedure originally used for the hysterectomy. A woman should discuss with her surgeon the need for continued Pap smear screening. Interestingly, pelvic exam is not considered sensitive or specific enough to serve as a screening tool for ovarian cancer, although it remains a common method for detecting this problem. Other detection methods for ovarian cancer include transvaginal or transabdominal ultrasound, color flow Doppler, and a blood test for the CA-125 antigen (Martin, 2004).

4.21   My doctor is recommending a hysterectomy. Should I have my ovaries removed, too?

This is a personal decision based on multiple factors including age, risk of ovarian cancer, risk of other diseases associated with hormones produced by the ovaries, current presence or absence of menopause, physician recommendation and rationale, and patient preference. A woman should discuss with her physician the risks and benefits of having her ovaries removed.

4.22   I have heard there is a new blood test for ovarian cancer. Does it work?

A blood test is available that detects the presence of CA-125, a tumor marker used to detect and monitor the presence of ovarian cancer. However, CA-125 is only found in some types of epithelial ovarian cancer. It is detected in approximately 80% of patients with ovarian cancer. Other tumor markers may exist as well. Lactic acid dehydrogenase, human chorionic gonadotropin, and alpha-fetoprotein are found in germ cell tumors, but their use in epithelial ovarian cancer is not well established. Carcinoembryonic antigen (CEA) levels are likely to be elevated in advanced and bulky disease, but CEA is considered a nonspecific marker and may be elevated in the presence of other types of cancer. Newer research studies using protein patterns, elevated lysophosphatidic acid levels, and decreased epidermal growth factor receptors all have shown improved sensitivity over CA-125 for ovarian cancer detection. Nevertheless, these tests only have been used in small research studies and are not widely available. Genetic counseling for women who are known to carry the *BRCA1* or *BRCA2* gene, and are subsequently at increased risk for breast and ovarian cancers, is an increasing focus as well (Meunier, 2005).

4.23   What are the risk factors for and symptoms of ovarian cancer?

Risk factors for ovarian cancer include age (usually older than 50); nulliparity; first birth after the age of 35; obesity; family history of ovarian cancer; personal history of endometrial, breast, or colon cancer; the use of estrogen-only hormone replacement; and European or North American descent. Although infertility treatment has not been proven to increase a woman's risk of ovarian cancer, anecdotal reports seem to suggest a link. This may be because of the underlying cause of infertility or perhaps because of the infertility treatments themselves. Genetic presence of *BRCA1* mutation associated with breast cancer and polycystic ovarian disease leads to ovarian cancer development in 5%–10% of women (Roesser & Mullineaux, 2005). Researchers have associated the use of oral contraceptives, pregnancy, and breast-feeding with a lower risk of ovarian cancer.

Symptoms of ovarian cancer usually result from extension of the disease beyond the pelvis, because the ovary itself can become very large without producing symptoms. For that reason, symptoms often are nonspecific and include bloating, abdominal swelling, abdominal or pelvic pain, abdominal fullness, pelvic pressure, dyspepsia, anorexia, urinary frequency, and weight gain. Weight loss, nausea, vomiting, anorexia, and severe pain are associated with advanced disease.

Q 4.24   Why is the mortality rate so high for ovarian cancer?

Mortality for ovarian cancer is linked to many factors. The most critical factor related to treatment outcome is the stage of the disease at the time of diagnosis. Unfortunately, many women with ovarian cancer are unaware of their disease until it has advanced. Initial treatment results vary based on the stage of disease at diagnosis. Metastasis usually occurs through direct extension of disease and hematologic spread. Sadly, although many chemotherapy agents have been used in treating recurrent ovarian cancer, response rates usually are poor.

Q 4.25   What is the best treatment for ovarian cancer?

Options for treatment include surgery, chemotherapy, and radiation therapy. Treatment decisions depend on the stage of disease. Total abdominal hysterectomy and oophorectomy and other surgical techniques are used for treatment and for the detection of metastatic disease. Patients may undergo total abdominal and pelvic radiation or intraperitoneal radiation if minimal residual disease exists postoperatively. Combination chemotherapy with a taxane and a cisplatin- or carboplatin-based combination is considered standard treatment for more extensive disease. Neoadjuvant treatment aimed at reducing tumor burden preoperatively is now an option. Ovarian cancer recurs in up to 80% of women. Clinical trials and treatment approaches continue to evolve (Martin, 2004).

Summary

 4.26   What are the key questions I should ask my doctor in relation to these types of cancer?

Key points of concern for women to discuss with their physicians include the woman's individual risk factors, appropriate screening and early detection methods, and lifestyle management and cancer prevention. If a woman is diagnosed with a gynecologic malignancy, questions will focus on tumor type and stage, treatment options, potential for clinical trials, insurance coverage, and sources of support during treatment. Once treatment has begun, women should regularly discuss side effects and their management, disease response to therapy, emotional and personal issues related to the adjustments demanded by cancer and its treatment, and general health. If cancer treatment is successful and a woman is in remission, questions will focus on appropriate follow-up and monitoring, long-term side effects, and ongoing support for the woman and her significant others. Throughout the process, honest communication is a vital part of diagnosis, treatment, and health.

4.27   What side effects of treatment do women undergoing treatment for gynecologic cancer commonly experience?

Side effects will vary with each treatment modality. Because surgery, radiation therapy, and chemotherapy all can be used for various stages of cervical, uterine, or ovarian cancer, some side effects can be generalized.

In general, surgical side effects include pain and the potential for wound complications and infection. Radiation therapy may cause skin irritation and site-specific difficulties such as vaginal dryness or diarrhea. Because most gynecologic treatment regimens involve combination chemotherapy, side effects most likely will include nausea and vomiting, potential for hair loss, fatigue, potential for infection, and peripheral neuropathies. The physician will discuss specific regimens and will provide a more detailed discussion of side effects. Additionally, changes in body image, altered hormonal balance, and other factors place women undergoing treatment at risk for depression, weight gain or loss resulting from alterations in diet, changes in role patterns and relationships, and changes in sleep patterns.

Q 4.28   What support organizations exist to assist patients and families?

Multiple support groups exist to support women with cancer and women with each specific diagnosis. Medical institutions and national groups such as the American Cancer Society and the National Cancer Coalition may host support groups. Programs such as the American Cancer Society's "I Can Cope" and "Look Good . . . Feel Better" are designed for patients with any cancer diagnosis and are a great source of emotional support for patients and families. Multiple resources for information and support are available on the Internet as well.

References

Jemal, A., Siegel, R., Ward, E., Murray, T., Xu, J., Smigal, C., et al. (2006). Cancer statistics, 2006. *CA: A Cancer Journal for Clinicians, 56,* 106–130.

Martin, V. (2004). Gynecological malignancies. In C. Varricchio (Ed.), *A cancer source book for nurses* (8th ed., pp. 295–307). Sudbury, MA: Jones and Bartlett.

Meunier, J. (2005, March). *GYN cancer: Current treatments and future possibilities.* Presented at the 15th annual Current Issues in Oncology Care Conferences, Lansing, MI.

Program for Appropriate Technology in Health. (2001). *Cervical cancer prevention fact sheet.* Retrieved June 25, 2005, from http://www.path.org/files/RH_fs_risk_factors.pdf

Roesser, K., & Mullineaux, L. (2005). *Genetic testing and hereditary cancer: Implications for nurses.* Pittsburgh, PA: Oncology Education Services.

Spinelli, A., Whitaker, L., & Birk, C. (2003, May). *Update in gynecologic oncology.* Instructional session presented at the Oncology Nursing Society 28th Annual Congress, Denver, CO.

Resources

American Cancer Society: www.cancer.org
Methodist Hospital System: www.methodisthealth.com/health/gynonc/uterine.htm
National Cancer Coalition: www.nationalcancercoalition.org
National Cancer Institute: www.cancer.gov
National Cervical Cancer Coalition: www.nccc-online.org
National Ovarian Cancer Coalition: www.ovarian.org
Oncology Nursing Society: www.ons.org

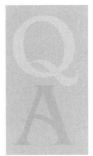

Chapter 5

Lung Cancer

Kelly J. Damman, RN, OCN®

Background

Q 5.1 What causes lung cancer?

Although multiple risk factors exist, the use of tobacco is the number-one cause of lung cancer. Approximately 90% of lung cancer cases are related to tobacco use. Nonsmokers also are at risk for developing lung cancer when they breathe tobacco smoke from smokers. Other contributing factors for lung cancer include extensive exposure to asbestos, diesel fuel, or radon, history of tuberculosis (TB), and possibly long-term exposure to air pollution (Alberg & Samet, 2003).

Q 5.2 Can lung cancer be prevented? If so, how?

Lung cancer is one of the few preventable cancers. The best lung cancer prevention tool is for people to never start smoking. For smokers, prevention requires quitting the habit. Other prevention tools include being aware of one's environment and avoiding exposure to secondhand smoke, radon, radiation, asbestos, diesel fuel, and air pollution. Lung cancer awareness is the key (Alberg & Samet, 2003).

Q 5.3 I have heard that there are different types of lung cancer. Can you describe these to me?

Two types of lung cancer exist: non-small cell lung cancer (NSCLC) and small cell lung cancer (SCLC). Although they both are types of lung cancer, they are very different.

NSCLC is the most common type of lung cancer; it accounts for approximately 80% of the cases. NSCLC is further categorized into subtypes: adenocarcinoma, squamous cell, and large cell. NSCLC usually is associated with smoking, passive smoke exposure, and environmental factors such as radon, asbestos, and air pollution. SCLC (sometimes called oat cell cancer) accounts for approximately 20% of lung cancer cases and almost always is related to smoking. SCLC is fast growing and very likely to spread outside of the lung early in the disease process (Houlihan, 2004).

Q 5.4 **How many Americans are diagnosed with lung cancer each year, and how does this compare with other cancers?**

More than 170,000 Americans are diagnosed with lung cancer annually. Lung cancer ranks third among the most commonly diagnosed cancers, behind breast and prostate cancers. The American Cancer Society (ACS, 2006) estimated that 174,470 new lung cancer cases will be diagnosed in 2006, along with 214,640 new breast cancer cases and 234,460 new prostate cancer cases. Additionally, ACS estimated 20,180 ovarian cancer cases, 62,190 cases of melanoma, and 106,680 new cases of colon cancer in 2006.

Q 5.5 **I'm confused. I hear so much in the media about women and breast cancer, but now I hear that more women die from lung cancer each year. Is this true?**

Yes. According to the ACS (2006), 72,130 women will die from lung cancer in 2006. This number is steadily rising. In comparison, 40,970 women will die from breast cancer. Unfortunately, the media coverage of cancer sometimes is misleading.

Risk Factors

Q 5.6 **What are the risk factors for developing lung cancer?**

The most obvious and preventable risk factor for lung cancer is tobacco use. More than 90% of all lung cancer cases are attributed to exposure to tobacco smoke. The longer a person smokes and the more he or she smokes, the higher the risk becomes.

Other risk factors include occupational and environmental exposures to tobacco smoke, radon, asbestos, diesel fuel, radiation, and air pollution. The genetic risk for lung cancer is being studied and is not well understood at this time. Recent research shows that women may be more likely to develop lung cancer than men; however, the reason is not clearly understood. Some feel that this is because the number of female smokers is on the rise, whereas the number of male smokers is on the decline (Alberg & Samet, 2003).

 5.7 What is the relationship between lung cancer and smoking?

Smoking is the number-one cause of lung cancer, and the best way to prevent lung cancer is to refrain from smoking. One must keep in mind that it is never too late to stop smoking. The longer people smoke and the more they smoke, the greater their chances of developing lung cancer. Smoking damages the lungs, and it is not until smoking ceases that the lung tissues can begin to heal.

Although smoking cessation will not guarantee that a person will never get lung cancer, it significantly reduces the risk of developing the disease. Past smokers never can reduce their lung cancer risk to that of a nonsmoker (Alberg & Samet, 2003).

5.8 My doctor asked me about my smoking "pack-year" history. What is this?

This is a mathematical calculation taking into consideration the number of years the patient has smoked multiplied by the number of packs of cigarettes smoked per day (1 pack per day x 20 years = 20 pack-year history). Healthcare professionals determine a person's lung cancer risk by using this calculation. The higher the pack-year history, the higher one's risk for developing lung cancer at some time in his or her life (Alberg & Samet, 2003).

5.9 I stopped smoking more than 20 years ago. Why did I get lung cancer?

Although smoking cessation reduces a person's risk for lung cancer, once a person smokes, his or her risk never goes back to that of someone who has never smoked. For smokers who quit, in 15 years, their risk of lung cancer is 2 times that of a nonsmoker, rather than 10 times if they had continued smoking. Other environmental or hereditary factors also may need to be considered in determining why a person developed lung cancer (Alberg & Samet, 2003).

5.10 Why do nonsmokers get lung cancer?

Research is ongoing to attempt to answer this question; however, researchers may never know for sure. Approximately 16% of lung cancers occur in people who have never smoked. Healthcare professionals also know that passive smoke exposure increases the risk of a nonsmoker developing lung cancer. In fact, nonsmokers who are married to a smoker have a 30% higher risk of developing lung cancer than that of spouses of a nonsmoker (Alberg & Samet, 2003).

Other possible reasons for nonsmokers getting lung cancer have to do with other lung cancer risk factors, such as exposure to radon, asbestos, or diesel fuel, and previous lung disease, such as TB. The relationship of genetics is not well understood at this time (Alberg & Samet, 2003).

Detection

5.11   What are the symptoms of lung cancer?

Lung cancer has many symptoms, but they are not readily recognized because they often are mistaken for a cold or pneumonia. Because of this, lung cancer often is diagnosed after it already has spread.

The National Cancer Institute (1999) noted that some common symptoms include persistent cough or change in cough; shortness of breath; tiredness; blood in the sputum; pain in the chest, shoulder, upper back, or arm (sometimes aggravated by a deep breath); repeated episodes of pneumonia or bronchitis; unexplained weight loss or loss of appetite; unexplained hoarseness or wheezing; swelling of the neck or face; and unexplained fever.

5.12   Because lung cancer is so common, why don't we all get screened for it as we do for colon and breast cancers?

Although it seems sensible to be screened for lung cancer, research has not shown that screening for lung cancer improves disease survival. Another consideration is the method by which screening should be done and the risks involved with that method.

Ongoing studies are looking at screening high-risk individuals with a computed tomography (CT) scan versus chest x-ray. A CT scan is able to detect lung tumors, but it also will detect other noncancerous conditions. The results of the screening CT scan often lead to further testing that otherwise would not have been necessary.

Sometimes a lung biopsy is necessary to determine whether the suspicious finding is cancerous. A lung biopsy is very different from a breast or colon biopsy. A lung biopsy can result in difficulty breathing, bleeding, air in the lung, and other potentially life-threatening complications. With all of this in mind, the decision to screen all Americans for lung cancer has not been well-accepted and will not be until some definitive evidence shows that it saves lives (Bach, Kelley, Tate, & McCrory, 2003).

5.13   How is lung cancer detected and diagnosed?

Healthcare providers detect lung cancer by plain chest x-ray and CT scans, and they diagnose the disease by a tissue biopsy of the suspicious area. The majority of lung cancers are detected incidentally when a person has a medical evaluation for a different problem. A routine chest x-ray, done in preparation for another procedure, may detect a tumor that otherwise would not have been found.

Diagnosis may take place via a lung biopsy done with CT guidance, in the operating room when surgery is being done, or via a bronchoscopy procedure. Physicians can make a diagnosis only by obtaining a piece of tissue and having it examined under the microscope (Alliance for Lung Cancer Advocacy, Support, and Education [ALCASE], 1999).

5.14   What does my doctor mean when he says my lung cancer needs to be "staged"?

In order to decide the best way to treat any kind of cancer, doctors must determine the "stage." Healthcare professionals must first get an overall look at the extent of the person's disease. Once they know the size of the tumor, its location, and whether it has spread to nearby lymph nodes or distant organs, they can develop an individualized treatment plan. Staging determines whether the cancer can be surgically removed.

NSCLC is staged according to the American Joint Committee on Cancer staging criteria (Greene et al., 2002). These criteria take into account the size of the primary tumor (T), spread to regional lymph nodes (N), and distant metastasis (M). Furthermore, T can range from 1–4, based on the size of the tumor, its location, and whether it invades any nearby structures. N can range from 1–3, based on which lymph nodes are affected and on which side of the chest they are located. M refers to distant spread of the disease, or spread to the opposite lung or a different lobe of the same lung. Once the TNM is established, physicians can determine the stage grouping according to the TNM subset.

Lung cancer ranges from stage I through stage IV, with I being the earliest stage and IV the most advanced. Surgery usually is considered for stages I, II, and sometimes III, depending on the patient. Examples of staging are

- Stage I: No spread beyond the location of the primary tumor (T1–2, N0, M0)
- Stage II: Spread to lymph nodes in the lungs only, or a larger tumor with no nodes involved (T1–3, N0–1, M0)
- Stage III: Spread to lymph nodes but not to distant sites. It also can be a tumor that invades thoracic structures but does not involve the lymph nodes (T1–4, N0–3, M0).
- Stage IV: Spread to other parts of the body or other lobes of the same lung (T1–4, N0–3, M1).

Healthcare providers can determine the stage noninvasively by x-rays and scans or invasively by a surgical procedure. The noninvasive staging workup for lung cancer might include a chest x-ray, CT scan of the chest and abdomen, bone scan, CT or magnetic resonance imaging of the brain, or a positron-emission tomography scan. Surgical staging usually comes after the noninvasive staging has been completed and does not indicate that the cancer has spread to distant organs. This involves examining the lungs and lymph nodes in the chest during a surgical procedure.

During surgery, physicians will excise the cancer and some nearby lymph nodes, which a pathologist will then examine under a microscope. This procedure determines the specific type of tumor and whether the cancer involves any of the lymph nodes. Sometimes, an abnormality on a scan will prove not to be cancerous once examined under the microscope. This helps to support the importance of using both invasive and noninvasive techniques, if appropriate, when staging lung cancer (ALCASE, 1999).

Treatment

Q 5.15   What treatments currently are available for lung cancer?

Multiple treatments are available for lung cancer. The treatment of choice is surgery when the cancer is detected before it has spread to other parts of the body. Other treatment options include chemotherapy and radiation therapy. Some clinical trials also are looking at newer ways to treat lung cancer with agents that affect only the cancer cells.

Surgery is used to remove the cancer. Lung cancer surgery may involve removal of the tumor itself, the lobe of the lung, or the entire lung.

Chemotherapy is the use of chemicals to kill cancer cells. Chemotherapy kills cancer cells but also kills normal cells. When chemotherapy kills normal cells, patients experience side effects. Chemotherapy commonly is given intravenously but also may be in the form of a pill.

Radiation therapy is the use of high-energy rays to kill cancer cells. Radiation is aimed at a specific area and only affects the treated area, unlike chemotherapy, which goes throughout the body.

Sometimes healthcare providers use a combined treatment approach to treat lung cancer. Many patients will receive a combination of all three modalities in managing their individual case (National Cancer Institute, 1999).

5.16   Can't the lung cancer simply be removed surgically?

Surgical removal depends on the type, location, and extent of the tumor. When the tumor is large and invades other nearby organ structures, it may not be possible for the surgeon to cut out the tumor. Removing the tumor may require the surgeon to cut a major blood vessel or organ, and this could be life threatening to the patient.

Some types of lung cancers, such as small cell, are so aggressive that surgery is not considered. Small cell is always considered a systemic disease at the time of diagnosis because most cancers of this type will have spread to the lymph nodes in the chest or other organs. In this case, surgery could not remove all of the cancer; thus, surgery would not be attempted (ALCASE, 1999).

5.17   Why did my friend have her entire lung removed when she had lung cancer, whereas I only had to have a lobe of my lung removed?

The extent of surgery depends on the location and size of the tumor. The goal of surgery is to completely remove the cancerous mass. When the tumor involves only one lobe of the lung, the individual lobe may be removed (lobectomy). However, when the tumor is large or extends to other lobes of the lung, the entire lung may need to be removed (pneumonectomy) in order to remove all of the cancer. In some cases, the surgeon may have a personal preference to remove the lung instead of just the lobe. The individual health status of the patient also must be considered in planning a surgical approach (ALCASE, 1999).

5.18   How long is the recovery period following lung cancer surgery?

A common misconception exists about recovering from lung surgery. Many do not realize that it takes a number of months to fully recover from lung surgery. In addition, the person's body must compensate for the part of the lung that was removed by surgery. Eventually, the person will get back to his or her normal activity level, but it may be six or more months before he or she feels normal again.

5.19   Will I look or feel any different after my lung is removed?

Chances are good that a patient will look exactly the same after his or her lung is removed. When the lung is removed, the other chest organs shift over to the center of the chest and fill in the empty spaces. Luckily, people have the rib cage to maintain the shape of the chest and protect the chest cavity from injury. Eventually, breathing also should return to a normal state (ALCASE, 1999).

5.20   Why didn't my oncologist offer me chemotherapy or radiation therapy after my surgery to remove my lung cancer? I feel like my doctor is withholding life-saving treatment from me.

In this case, it sounds as though the physician detected and removed the cancer at an early stage (stage I or II). The standard treatment for early-stage lung cancer once was surgical removal, followed by close observation. Chemotherapy and radiation were saved for later use if the cancer recurred. Within the past few years, newer studies have shown that adding chemotherapy after surgical removal offers a small survival benefit. However, radiation rarely is used when the disease has been completely resected. Physicians must heavily weigh the side effects of chemotherapy and radiation therapy when using these treatments in patients who have no evidence of cancer at the time of treatment (Domont, Soria, & Le Chevalier, 2005).

Q 5.21 **Since taking lung cancer chemotherapy treatment, I have numb hands and feet. What is this, and how long will it last?**

This situation can occur when a patient has received a type of drug referred to as a "taxane." This family of drugs has a peculiar side effect of peripheral neuropathy. Peripheral neuropathy occurs when the nerves in the hands and feet are damaged in the process of the chemotherapy doing its job to kill the cancer cells. This usually is reversible but may take a number of months to completely subside. Patients should keep their physicians informed as to the status of their neuropathy because some medications can be considered if the symptoms become too uncomfortable (ALCASE, 1999).

Q 5.22 **After my friend was diagnosed with lung cancer, she also was diagnosed with brain and liver cancers. Why did she get three cancers?**

Chances are that she does not have three cancers but that her lung cancer has spread to her liver and brain. These are common sites to which lung cancer tends to spread. If she is unsure of her situation, she should ask her physician to clarify this.

Q 5.23 **I have lung cancer that has spread to my liver. Why won't the doctors do surgery to remove the cancer?**

Research has shown that once a tumor has metastasized, the disease has become more aggressive and is harder to manage and treat. Although it may be possible to do surgery to remove the cancer, healthcare professionals know that this would not provide a cure, and it may not lengthen or provide additional quality to a patient's life, either.

Depending on the area of metastasis, the tumor may be inoperable, or multiple areas of spread may exist. Finally, the surgery itself may be too dangerous for a patient to survive because of factors such as age or underlying health status. In many cases, the surgical removal of the metastasis will not improve overall survival; thus, surgery is not a viable option.

Q 5.24 **Is lung cancer "curable"?**

This is a good question and is sometimes difficult to answer. Early detection and treatment of lung cancer offer the best chance for a "cure." All early-stage cases (stage I or II) should be treated with a curative intent. When lung cancer has spread, the possibility of cure is limited. It is known that 85% of those with lung cancer die from the disease, but 13% are cured. This demonstrates that healthcare professionals are not finding lung cancer early enough to offer a cure. Most think of "cure" as occurring when one is alive without evidence of the cancer for five years after completing treatment (Alberts, 2003).

5.25   What should I expect after my treatment is completed? Will I still need to see a doctor or have x-rays taken?

It is extremely important for patients to maintain timely follow-up with a physician after the diagnosis of lung cancer, even if they are done with treatments. Lung cancer comes back in many cases, and the best weapon to have available is early detection. Patients should have a chest x-ray every few months for the first few years after being diagnosed with lung cancer, then every six months for a couple of years, and then annually at their doctor's discretion. Along with the x-ray is the need for a physical examination by a physician at these same intervals.

Patients should maintain close contact with a physician so that any abnormalities can be promptly detected and appropriate action taken. Some physicians may perform CT scans as they continue to monitor for any evidence of lung cancer recurrence (Colice, Rubins, & Unger, 2003).

5.26   Why should someone take part in a research study for lung cancer treatment?

Many reasons exist for anyone who has cancer to take part in a research study. Medical professionals know what they know today because of research that was done in the past. Without research, none of the treatments that are available today would exist.

Many patients participate in research not for themselves but for those who will come later. They may want to further science and help others to have a better chance for cure than they do. For some, the study may offer the only opportunity to receive a new experimental treatment. For others, they may feel that the side effects of a new treatment sound milder than those of the standard treatment, so they decide to give the new treatment a try. This is an individual treatment decision, but healthcare providers encourage people to consider taking part in a clinical trial if they qualify for one (ALCASE, 1999).

5.27 **Why should I take any treatment for my lung cancer? I did this to myself by smoking for all those years; plus, the cancer eventually is going to end my life.**

First of all, patients should not think that they did this to themselves. As previously discussed, many reasons can cause people to get lung cancer. Despite the fact that a person smoked for years, he or she still deserves treatment and the best quality of life possible.

The treatments for lung cancer are very well tolerated and are given in a number of different ways so that patients can maintain *quality* of life as well as *quantity* of life. A person's prognosis depends on how much the cancer has spread. A doctor would not have recommended a treatment if he or she felt it were not in the patient's best interest. People should discuss their concerns with their physicians.

5.28 **Why isn't there more in the media about lung cancer?**

Good question. Many people look down upon those with lung cancer. Lung cancer carries a stigma that "you gave yourself the disease, and now you must suffer the consequences." Some other cancers and diseases have an emotional pull because the disease occurred as a result of nothing the people did to themselves. The truth is that many cases of lung cancer occur in lifelong nonsmokers.

5.29 **I have heard about support groups for patients with lung cancer. Should I join one?**

The decision to join a support group is a very individual one. A support group can provide a forum where patients can get to know others who can relate to what they are experiencing. Some feel a sense of comfort and relief when they can talk to others who have walked in their shoes. Support groups also may offer educational programs for participants. Patients may want to investigate the group before joining and set some goals for what they expect to gain from participation.

5.30 **I see so much on television about resources for breast cancer. Are there any resources available specifically for lung cancer?**

Unfortunately, far fewer resources are available specifically for patients with lung cancer when compared with other cancers. The Lung Cancer Alliance is an excellent resource for patients who need lung cancer information and support. The Lung Cancer Alliance can be reached at www.lungcanceralliance.org or by calling 800-298-2436.

Another excellent lung cancer resource is www.lungcancer.org and its program "It's Time to Focus on Lung Cancer." They also have a toll-free information line, which is available at 877-646-LUNG. Until the medical community can raise the awareness of lung cancer, and get people to understand that lung cancer can be prevented and that not all who get lung cancer are smokers, healthcare professionals will continue to face an uphill battle when it comes to lung cancer resources.

References

Alberg, A.J., & Samet, J.M. (2003). Epidemiology of lung cancer. *Chest, 123*(Suppl. 1), 21S–49S.

Alberts, W.M. (2003). Lung cancer guidelines. *Chest, 123*(Suppl. 1), 1S–2S.

Alliance for Lung Cancer Advocacy, Support, and Education. (1999). *The lung cancer manual.* Vancouver, WA: Author.

American Cancer Society. (2006). *Cancer facts and figures, 2006.* Atlanta, GA: Author.

Bach, P.B., Kelley, M.J., Tate, R.C., & McCrory, D.C. (2003). Screening for lung cancer: A review of the current literature. *Chest, 123*(Suppl. 1), 72S–82S.

Colice, G.L., Rubins, J., & Unger, M. (2003). Follow-up and surveillance of the lung cancer patient following curative-intent therapy. *Chest, 123*(Suppl. 1), 272S–283S.

Domont, J., Soria, J.C., & Le Chevalier, T. (2005). Adjuvant chemotherapy in early-stage non-small cell lung cancer. *Seminars in Oncology, 32,* 279–283.

Greene, F.L., Page, D.L., Fleming, I.D., Fritz, A., Balch, C.M., Haller, D.G., et al. (2002). *AJCC cancer staging manual* (6th ed.). New York: Springer-Verlag.

Houlihan, N.G. (2004). Overview. In N.G. Houlihan (Ed.), *Site-specific cancer series: Lung cancer* (pp. 1–5). Pittsburgh, PA: Oncology Nursing Society.

National Cancer Institute. (1999). *What you need to know about lung cancer.* Bethesda, MD: Author.

Resources

American Cancer Society: www.cancer.org
Lung Cancer Alliance: www.lungcanceralliance.org
Lungcancer.org: www.lungcancer.org
National Cancer Institute: www.cancer.gov

Chapter 6

Fibromyalgia Syndrome

Sarah McGrew, BSN, RN

Background

6.1 **What is fibromyalgia syndrome (FMS)?**

FMS is a common condition associated with widespread musculoskeletal pain, fatigue, and excessive tenderness to pressure on 11 of 18 tender points. Diseases that have symptoms similar to FMS, such as hypothyroidism, chronic fatigue syndrome, allergies, irritable bowel and bladder syndromes, restless leg syndrome, and certain rheumatic conditions, may be present. It is possible to have another condition along with FMS.

The American College of Rheumatology (ACR) criteria developed in 1990 for FMS include widespread body pain in all four quadrants lasting longer than three consecutive months and the presence of pain in 11 out of 18 anatomically defined tender points (Wolfe et al., 1990). Goldenberg (2004) noted that these criteria provide a sensitivity and specificity of nearly 85% in differentiating between FMS and other forms of chronic musculoskeletal pain. However, patients often experience pain in other locations; Clauw (2001) estimated that half of the individuals with a diagnosis of FMS do not fit the ACR criteria.

Both Clauw (2001) and Goldenberg (2004) suggested that when FMS is suspected, an appropriate workup should include a thorough history, including sleep and mood disorders, and a physical exam. Laboratory testing should include a complete blood count, erythrocyte sedimentation rate or C-reactive protein, thyroid-stimulating hormone, and liver function tests.

6.2 **Who gets FMS and why?**

No one knows for sure why FMS develops in some people, although a genetic link is suspected. Russell and Iyengar (2004) reported that approximately 30% of people with FMS can identify another family member with a similar condition or with a diagnosis of FMS. This syndrome affects at least 2% of the general population in the United States, and this figure seems to be the same worldwide. Approximately 90% of the people affected are women. Patients usually receive diagnoses between the ages of 45 and 60, although some people claim to have had symptoms since they were children.

6.3   What confounds the diagnosis of FMS?

FMS is difficult to diagnose because no cost-effective lab tests or x-rays are available to confirm the clinical findings, and physicians must consider other conditions before making the diagnosis. An early and accurate diagnosis will save the patient time, money, and unnecessary distress. However, many patients go for months or years before FMS is diagnosed. Although symptoms of FMS have long been reported in the medical literature, FMS was not considered to be a disease until 1990, when the aforementioned diagnostic criteria were developed. Research published by Desmeules et al. (2003) conclusively found abnormalities in the cerebrospinal fluid of people with FMS, although obtaining cerebrospinal fluid to confirm a diagnosis carries too many risks to be used as a general diagnostic tool.

Symptoms

6.4   What are tender points?

Tender points are specific areas on the body that hurt when pressure is applied. Certain tender points are used primarily for diagnostic purposes; people with FMS usually also hurt in places that are not considered diagnostic tender points. Some people use the words "tender points" and "trigger points" to mean the same thing, whereas others consider trigger points to be places in muscles that hurt. An experienced physician may inject tender/trigger points with local anesthesia when other treatments do not relieve the pain.

6.5   What other symptoms typically accompany a diagnosis of FMS?

Some other symptoms are very commonly found in people with FMS. They include morning stiffness, fatigue, headaches, sleep disturbances, depression, anxiety, chest wall pain, irritable bowel and bladder, and numbness and tingling in the extremities. Not being able to think clearly, or "fibro fog," also is a frequent complaint, as are cold intolerance, dizziness, and allergies.

6.6   What is happening in my body to make me feel so bad?

Research is ongoing to determine exactly what is happening in the brain and body when a person has symptoms of FMS. A malfunction in the stress response system and neuroendocrine function is suspected (Goldenberg, 2004). Abnormal levels of neurotransmitters, such as dopamine, serotonin, and norepinephrine and neurochemicals such as substance P have been found in the blood and cerebrospinal fluid of people with FMS, which places FMS within a model of central nervous system sensitization. People with FMS typically experience pain from stimuli that would not feel painful to others, and the perception of pain continues after the source of pain is removed. They also usually cannot tolerate pain for as long. These findings are known as allodynia and hyperalgesia.

6.7   Does FMS ever go away?

FMS is a chronic condition and cannot be completely cured. However, it can be successfully treated. This is best accomplished when the person with FMS has been educated about the disease, is actively involved in his or her treatment, and works with a treatment team (which may include a family physician, rheumatologist, nurse, physical therapist, psychologist, massage therapist, and others) that is supportive and well informed about FMS. A caring family and/or group of friends also are very helpful to the person with FMS.

6.8   Is depression a cause of FMS?

Healthcare professionals used to consider depression to be a cause of FMS, but this has been disproved. Clauw (2001) reported that roughly 40% of people with FMS have depression; this figure is similar to the number of people diagnosed with rheumatoid arthritis who also have depression. However, 40% is a significant number of people, and depression and anxiety are associated with FMS. Treating depression often is part of the treatment of FMS. This treatment can include exercise, medications, and cognitive behavioral therapy.

Q 6.9 Why am I forgetful? Is that related?

As mentioned in Question 5, impaired thinking often is a complaint of people with FMS. The reason behind this is not clearly understood, but using some simple techniques can help people with FMS to boost memory. One suggestion is to get into the habit of putting commonly used items such as car keys in the same place after each use. Writing down information as it is received can be helpful. People with FMS can provide cues for themselves by keeping a "to-do" list. Both reducing stress levels and treating depression can help to limit confusion. Staying physically and mentally active also is a useful way to limit absentmindedness.

Q 6.10 Does stress make FMS worse?

Many people with FMS report that stress increases their symptoms. The causes of "stress" are different for different people. They might include physical stress such as too much activity, illness, or injury. Emotional stressors such as worries about relationships, finances, and employment also may increase the symptoms of FMS. Controlling stress with good coping strategies and balancing rest with activity can improve the symptoms of FMS.

Q 6.11 How can I learn to control my stress?

First, identify the symptoms of stress, and determine the cause. Symptoms of excessive stress may be substance abuse, trouble sleeping, over- or undereating, irritability, anxiety, and physical complaints such as fatigue, increased pain, and stomach upset. Relaxation exercises such as guided imagery and visualization are good ways to reduce stress. Meditation, sometimes also called "mindfulness," is another strategy to reduce stress. Different people relax in different ways; some might watch a funny movie, whereas others take a walk or talk to a friend. Individuals should find a strategy that works for them. If the first attempt does not help, try something else. They can seek support from someone they trust. Patients' healthcare providers may have some stress management resources to suggest, as well.

Q 6.12 How can I get a good night's sleep?

Sleep disturbances are very common among people with FMS and may increase the feelings of pain, tiredness, and difficulty concentrating. Different people have different experiences in regard to sleep; some have trouble falling asleep, whereas others wake early feeling exhausted. Sleep apnea, with heavy snoring and periods of no breathing, may be occurring and must be either ruled out or followed up with sleep studies. Techniques to get a good night's sleep include setting a regular bedtime with enough hours for sleep. A bedtime ritual, such as a warm bath or a cup of herbal tea, is helpful for some people. Others experience a sense of calm with meditation or prayer before getting into bed. A peaceful bedroom (not too hot or cold, with little light) and a comfortable mattress also are conducive to restful sleep. Finally, keeping the bedroom as a place for sleep and intimate activities only (and not a place for talking on the phone or paying bills) helps to induce and maintain a good night's sleep.

Q __6.13__   **What can I do to help family members understand?**

It may be difficult for family and friends to understand this condition because a person with FMS usually does not look sick. Significant others may have expectations that are no longer realistic. Explaining feelings and thoughts in a way the other person can understand, by saying "I feel" instead of "you make me feel," can help to open the doors of communication. It is important to remember that the changes people with FMS experience affect family members, too. They may be dealing with financial stressors because of loss of employment income and additional costs of medical care, a change in intimate relations, or a parent who is no longer able to manage responsibilities or attend family events. Supporting each other by open communication is a way for family members to understand each other's concerns. A spouse may accompany the patient to a physician's appointment or to a support group for people with FMS. This may help to increase awareness and change any unrealistic expectations.

Interventions

Q __6.14__   **What medicines are helpful and in what doses?**

According to Goldenberg (2004), tricyclic antidepressants (TCAs) taken one to three hours before bedtime have been shown to be the most effective treatment for FMS. Dosage of these may include amitriptyline, nortriptyline (Pamelor®, Mallinckrodt, St. Louis, MO), and desipramine (Norpramin®, Aventis, Bridgewater, NJ), beginning at very low doses of 5–10 mg. These medications can be increased gradually by 5–10 mg every two weeks to obtain the most therapeutic dose while avoiding side effects. Ten to 30 mg of the muscle relaxant cyclobenzaprine (Flexeril®, McNeil, Fort Washington, PA) taken at bedtime also has proved effective.

Goldenberg, Burckhardt, and Crofford (2004) found modest evidence of the effectiveness of tramadol (Ultram®, Ortho-McNeil Pharmaceutical, Raritan, NJ) at a dose of 200–300 mg/day taken with or without acetaminophen. Moderate evidence exists to suggest that 20–80 mg of the selective serotonin reuptake inhibitor (SSRI) fluoxetine (Prozac®, Eli Lilly, Indianapolis, IN) may be effective in treating FMS. Dual reuptake inhibitors of serotonin and norepinephrine (SNRIs) such as venlafaxine (Effexor®, Wyeth, Philadelphia, PA) and duloxetine (Cymbalta®, Eli Lilly) also may be effective when taken at the recommended dosages for depression. These drugs may be used in conjunction with a TCA at bedtime for improved symptom control. Milnacipran® (Cypress Bioscience, San Diego, CA), a drug that inhibits equally the reuptake of both norepinephrine and serotonin, was effective in one randomized controlled trial. Phase III trials still are under way, although the drug is available in Europe. The anticonvulsant pregabalin (Lyrica®, Pfizer, New York, NY) was found effective at 450 mg/day in a single randomized controlled trial; gabapentin (Neurontin®, Pfizer) also is commonly used but has not been studied for FMS.

Goldenberg et al. (2004) found weak evidence for treatment with growth hormone except in a subset of patients with low growth hormone levels; they found no evidence for the effectiveness of opioids, steroids, nonsteroidal anti-inflammatory drugs, benzodiazepines or other hypnotics, melatonin, calcitonin, thyroid hormone, guaifenesin, dehydroepiandrosterone, or magnesium.

Clauw (2001) reported that trigger point injections, shots of anesthetic directly into painful muscles, may be used when FMS symptoms are not responding to more traditional treatments. However, Goldenberg et al. (2004) did not find any evidence for the effectiveness of trigger point injections.

Q 6.15   What are the side effects of these medications?

The most common side effects of TCAs are blurred vision, dry mouth, orthostatic hypotension, sweating, weight gain, and morn-

ing grogginess. Tramadol may cause dizziness, headaches, grogginess, weakness, nausea, constipation, itching, and difficulty
breathing. The SSRIs may cause headaches, grogginess, dizziness,
nervousness, insomnia, constipation, dry mouth, and sexual side
effects. More common side effects from SNRIs are cough, diarrhea, constipation, dizziness, dry mouth, fever, frequent urination, headache, lack or loss of strength, anorexia, muscle aches,
nausea, drowsiness, sore throat, stuffy or runny nose, diapho-
resis, insomnia, fatigue, weakness, vomiting, and weight loss.
Side effects from the anticonvulsants are not common but may
include drowsiness, headache, fatigue, blurred vision, tremor,
anxiety, and irregular eye movements. Trigger point injections
using local anesthetics may cause seizures, irregular heartbeats,
and bradycardia.

**6.16 What nonpharmacologic remedies are effective for managing symp-
toms of FMS?**

Goldenberg et al. (2004) found that cardiovascular exercise done
routinely, cognitive behavioral therapy, group patient education,
and combinations of these activities all had strong evidence as
effective nondrug treatments for FMS. Treatments with modest
evidence for effectiveness were strength training, acupuncture,
hypnotherapy, biofeedback, and medicinal baths (balneothera-
py). Weak evidence exists to suggest that chiropractic treatment,
manual and massage therapy, electrotherapy, and ultrasound may
improve symptoms. The authors did not find evidence to support
trigger point injections or flexibility exercises, but these may help
some patients.

People with FMS often use alternative remedies. When choosing
an alternative remedy, it is important to ask whether any studies
have been done on the treatment or whether the claims are just
stories from alleged sources. If studies have been done, was there
a control group, and was it a randomized controlled trial? Be wary
if a treatment claims to cure FMS; this is highly unlikely. Patients
should learn all they can about side effects of the remedy they are
considering, including "natural" and herbal products. Some can
be quite dangerous, particularly if patients are taking other medications. Patients should talk with their healthcare provider before
taking an herbal medicine or over-the-counter supplement and
always should report use of these substances when asked for a list
of their medications.

6.17   I have FMS. What can I do to help myself?

People with FMS can do many things to help themselves. They can be well informed about their condition and choose a supportive team of healthcare providers. They should consider themselves part of the healthcare team and communicate well with each care partner. FMS is different in different people, and each person's treatments should be the best "fit" for the individual. Patients should be open to trying new things but should critically evaluate treatments that have not yet been thoroughly studied. Patients should stay physically and mentally active, stay involved with friends and family, and believe in themselves. The Arthritis Self-Help Program (Stanford University), a patient education program available through the Arthritis Foundation, has been proved to reduce the discomfort associated with FMS and help participants to feel they have more control over the disease. To find local foundation chapters, call 800-283-7800, or visit the Foundation's Web site at www.arthritis.org.

6.18   I am too tired to exercise; can I try something else?

Moderate exercise is a cornerstone of treatment. Exercise can help to reduce fatigue, relieve depression, and improve sleep and fuzzy thinking. A person may be out of shape because he or she has been inactive for a long time; it will help to start out slowly.

Gentle stretching and strengthening with a modest walking program is a good place to start. Patients also might consider the Arthritis Foundation's Aquatic Program and Exercise Program. A physical therapist or exercise physiologist can provide specific suggestions.

6.19   What other strategies can be used to manage pain?

Other ways are available to manage pain in addition to exercise. Practicing relaxation exercises on a regular basis can reduce pain and anxiety. Some people find massage therapy extremely useful, whereas others swear by hot/cold treatments. Having a sense of humor also helps. Negative thinking patterns may be adding to physical and mental discomfort and can be treated through cognitive-behavioral therapy with a trained and licensed psychologist. Self-help books such as the Arthritis Foundation's (2001) *Guide to Good Living With Fibromyalgia* and the *Good Living With Fibromyalgia Workbook* (Afshar, 2002), both available from the Arthritis Foundation, may be useful.

6.20   Where can I turn for more information about FMS?

The Arthritis Foundation is an excellent source of information and may be able to help people find an exercise program and/or support group in their area. If these programs are not available nearby, this may be a good time to start one! The National Fibromyalgia Association has all kinds of useful information. See the list of resources at the end of this chapter for useful Web sites.

6.21   What is going on in the research world?

Research currently is being done on a wide variety of FMS symptoms and treatments. One area of study is the possibility that subsets of people with FMS may exist, some who are more likely to have depression and some who are more likely to have neurally mediated hypotension. Treatments may be developing to specifically treat people in those subgroups. Other studies are taking place on the topics of genetics, medications for patients with depression and pain or irritable bowel, medications such as ropinirole (Requip®, GlaxoSmithKline, Research Triangle Park, NC) and Milnacipran, the effects of stress on pain sensitivity, the relationship between irritable bowel and FMS, stress hormone studies, and sex-related determinants of pain. For more information on research, contact the National Institutes of Health, the Arthritis Foundation, or the National Fibromyalgia Association.

References

Afshar, B. (2002). *The good living with fibromyalgia workbook: Activities for a better life.* Atlanta, GA: Arthritis Foundation.

Arthritis Foundation. (2001). *Arthritis Foundation's guide to good living with fibromyalgia.* Atlanta, GA: Author.

Clauw, D. (2001). Fibromyalgia and diffuse pain syndromes. In J. Klippel, L. Crofford, J. Stone, & C. Weyand (Eds.), *Primer on the rheumatic diseases* (12th ed., pp. 188–193). Atlanta, GA: Arthritis Foundation.

Desmeules, J.A., Cedraschi, C., Rapiti, E., Baumgartner, E., Finckh, A., Cohen, P., et al. (2003). Neurophysiologic evidence for a central sensitization in patients with fibromyalgia. *Arthritis and Rheumatism, 48,* 1420–1429.

Goldenberg, D. (2004). Update on the treatment of fibromyalgia. *Bulletin on the Rheumatic Diseases, 53*(1). Retrieved July 31, 2005, from http://www.arthritis.org/research/Bulletin/Vol53No1/Introduction.asp

Goldenberg, D., Burckhardt, C., & Crofford, L. (2004). Management of fibromyalgia syndrome. *JAMA, 292,* 2388–2395.

Russell, J., & Iyengar, S. (2004). Is FM inherited? *Fibromyalgia Aware, 7,* 24–27.

Wolfe, F., Smythe, H.A., Yunus, M.B., Bennett, R.M., Bombardier, C., Goldenberg, D.L., et al., (1990). The American College of Rheumatology 1990 criteria for the classification of fibromyalgia: Report of the multicenter criteria committee. *Arthritis and Rheumatixm, 33,* 160–172.

Resources

Arthritis Foundation: www.arthritis.org
National Fibromyalgia Association: www.fmaware.org
National Institutes of Health: www.nih.gov

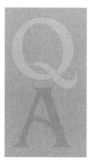

Chapter 7
Urinary Incontinence

Doreen A. White, BSN, RN, CWOCN

Background

Q 7.1 **At what point in the aging process may I expect urinary incontinence (UI)?**

UI can happen at any time in a person's life, but it is not a natural or inevitable outcome for women.

Q 7.2 **Is there a correlation between the onset of menopause and UI?**

No. UI is not a normal function of aging. It can happen at any age for a variety of reasons and may be temporary during a urinary tract infection (UTI), a vaginal infection or irritation, or constipation. Some medications may contribute to UI (Agency for Health Care Policy and Research [AHCPR], 1996c).

UI may be permanent if there is a weakness of the muscles holding the bladder in place, weakness of the sphincter muscles, with female hormone imbalances, with some neurologic disorders, and even with immobility (AHCPR, 1996b).

Q 7.3 **I only lose urine when I sneeze or cough. My friend can't make it to the bathroom in time as soon as she has the urge. Why are our symptoms different?**

Women can have different types of UI. In each case, specific treatments are available to improve their condition. Each woman should consult her healthcare provider for initial diagnosis and treatment recommendations.

Q 7.4   What are the different types of UI?

Three commonly recognized types of UI exist. *Urge* incontinence usually is associated with urine leakage when a person cannot get to the bathroom quickly enough, when he or she hears water running, or with other triggers. *Stress* incontinence usually is precipitated by exercise, sneezing, coughing, walking, or moving in a certain way. *Overflow* incontinence occurs when the bladder has not completely emptied. Frequently, the woman with this type of incontinence feels as if her bladder is still partly full even after urination. Overflow incontinence symptoms include a weak, dribbling urinary stream or loss of small amounts of urine both day and night. Finally, some people have *mixed* incontinence, meaning they experience a combination of two types of incontinence (AHCPR, 1996b).

Q 7.5   How can I approach my physician about my UI?

Directly. A physician will not be embarrassed. Physicians are concerned about their patients' health and well-being and can discuss treatment options with them. Many treatment options are available. If a person's physician offers only one suggestion, she should obtain a second opinion (AHCPR, 1996b).

Treatment

Q 7.6   Are there nonsurgical treatments for UI?

Yes. Nonsurgical treatments include exercises to improve muscle tone, electrical stimulation treatments, and medications to control UI. Specific nonsurgical treatments available to address UI problems are
- Bladder training—Involves resisting the urge to urinate, postponing urination, or urinating on a timetable
- Prescription medications
  - Stress incontinence: Pseudoephedrine—increases tension of the muscles of the bladder neck and urethra to retain urine
  - Urge incontinence
    * Imipramine (tricyclic antidepressant)—Causes bladder muscle to relax and the bladder neck to contract.
    * The following reduce smooth muscle spasms: Oxybutynin (anticholinergic/antispasmodic), tolterodine, dicyclomine, and hyoscyamine
- Pelvic muscle exercises—Repetitive exercise of specific perineal muscles

- Vaginal weight training—Holding small vaginal cones of increasing weights in the vagina to strengthen pelvic muscles
- Biofeedback—A signal display showing muscle effort giving a person information about the pelvic muscular activity
- Electrical stimulation—Applying an electric current to the pelvic structures and nerve supply to induce a therapeutic response

All may be options depending on the type of UI a person has (AHCPR, 1996a).

7.7 Is hormone replacement therapy (HRT) helpful with UI?

The bladder base, the urethra, and the vagina all originate from the same embryologic structure, which has high concentrations of estrogen receptors. Once menopause has occurred, these structures become estrogen depleted and weakened. Estrogen replacement plays a role in decreasing both UI and UTIs (Maloney, 2002). In postmenopausal women, HRT is being used to alleviate symptoms of UI. When using HRT, patients typically receive it in low concentrations through topical intravaginal creams, tablets, or rings (AHCPR, 1996a; Chiarelli, 2005).

7.8 What are the benefits of hormone replacement?

The use of HRT is controversial, and the reports of efficacy in providing relief to women with UI are mixed. Positive results have been reported with mild cases of stress incontinence. Because of the current controversy about HRT, all women need to discuss with their healthcare providers whether HRT is the proper approach for them (Newman, 2003).

7.9 Are there herbal remedies for UI treatment?

When UI occurs because of UTI, several herbs such as bayberry leaf and *Echinacea purpurea* have been cited as beneficial. Cranberry juice is an old standard and may be helpful (Gray, 2002). Because no general standards of quality exist for herbal substances in the United States, patients should obtain herbal preparations from reputable manufacturers. Patients always should consult their healthcare provider before using nonprescription products because interactions between prescription and nonprescription products may be detrimental to their overall health (Maloney, 2002).

7.10 Can certain medications complicate or worsen my UI?

Yes. Often, healthcare professionals prescribe these medications for conditions unrelated to UI. Typical classes of medications that can complicate or worsen UI are diuretics, sedatives, narcotics, antihistamines, anticholinergics, antipsychotics/antidepressants, and calcium channel blockers (AHCPR, 1996a; Doughty, 1991).

7.11   Are surgical treatments available for UI?

Yes. Surgical procedures may include correction of severely weakened pelvic muscles, enlargement of a small bladder to hold more urine, or return of the bladder neck to its proper position. A woman's incontinence type and her physician's recommendations will determine whether surgery is appropriate for her and, if so, the specific surgical procedure (AHCPR, 1996b).

7.12   What things can I try on my own to limit my UI?

First, women with UI should speak with their healthcare provider to determine the cause of their UI. Behavioral techniques such as bladder training and pelvic muscle exercises have proved useful for urge and stress incontinence. Patients can master these techniques using information and instruction provided by the healthcare provider.

7.13   My grandmother in the nursing home has UI. Is a urinary catheter the only option?

Other options are available besides a urinary catheter. Behavioral changes are appropriate to try if overflow incontinence is not the problem. An example is habit training. Here, the time a person goes to the toilet is matched to the person's voiding patterns. This involves timed, scheduled voiding at regular intervals, usually every two to three hours (AHCPR, 1996c).

7.14   Are there ways to keep my frail mother dry in her diapers?

A wide variety of incontinence products are on the market. Undergarments with full-length pads usually are held in place with waist straps. Adult pull-up disposable briefs have recently gained in popularity. Combination pad-pant systems provide security around the legs. The level of protection and absorption should dictate a person's choice.

7.15   Do the protective pads and diaper products on the market limit the perineal skin damage of UI?

Yes, if used correctly and changed regularly. The disposable products will wick the urine away from the skin into the middle of the incontinence brief or pad. The middle layers contain polymers that gel to prevent seepage. In all cases, these products require regular changing and perineal skin cleansing to prevent skin irritation and damage.

7.16 Are all these disposable diapers affecting our environment?

Disposable diapers make up the largest portion of absorbent hygiene products in use in North America. To meet this demand for disposable diapers in the United States, approximately a quarter of a million trees, equivalent to 1.3 million tons of wood pulp, are required annually. Most of this high-quality wood fiber then is dumped into landfills instead of being reclaimed. Recycling of this material currently is in use in Europe and Canada and is planned for use in California. In the recycling process, soiled diapers are brought to a processor and treated through a combination chemical/mechanical process. This results in a reduced amount of material sent to landfills and produces a stream of raw material that can be reused in nonfood products ranging from wallpaper to roof shingles (Chobanian, 2002).

7.17 Why is UI so damaging to perineal skin?

Normal skin is slightly acidic. The ammonia and urea in urine cause the skin to become more alkaline. This shift from acid to alkaline irritates skin, causing dermatitis. In addition, normal skin bacteria can increase in the presence of the excessive moisture arising from UI. This causes an increased incidence of skin infections such as *Candida albicans* (Doughty, 1991).

7.18 How do pelvic exercises help UI?

Pelvic floor muscle, or Kegel, exercises were introduced in 1948. Studies have shown Kegel exercises to be effective in the management of both urge and stress UI. To be successful, the individual must be instructed in identifying the correct muscle group and how to effectively contract that muscle group. The duration of contraction and number of repetitions are specific to the instructor and severity of the person's condition (Johnson, 2001).

7.19 How does biofeedback treatment work for UI?

This is a method to teach the person effective pelvic floor exercises. Small sensors close to the muscles being monitored measure the strength of the muscle contraction. The sensors record the muscle effort as a bar moving along a screen or an audible signal so the individual can see or hear how effectively she is contracting the particular muscle. Generally, the person reports back to the clinic weekly while continuing an established exercise regimen every day at home (Johnson, 2001).

7.20   Will high-impact aerobics cause me to have UI?

Information suggests that repetitive bouncing in activities such as running are most likely to provoke incontinence *if* that intensity exceeds a person's continence threshold. Congenital or hereditary factors such as muscle mass influence this threshold. Acquired factors such as injury during childbirth or certain medications can contribute to this outcome, as well (Nygaard, 2002).

7.21   How should I manage UI during intercourse?

Women should make sure their bladder and bowels are empty before intercourse. Use warmed lubricating gel and avoid positions that may cause urine leakage. Women with UI should share their concerns with their sexual partner instead of curtailing sexual intimacy. Also, women should consult their healthcare provider about what other options—surgical and nonsurgical—may be helpful for them (Weber, 2001).

7.22   Are there lifestyle changes to improve my UI?

First, women should manage their fluid intake while ensuring they maintain adequate fluid intake of at least six 8-ounce glasses of liquid, preferably water, every day. Adequate fluid intake prevents the urine from becoming highly concentrated. Highly concentrated urine can irritate the bladder and cause a sense of urgency or frequency. If nighttime incontinence is a problem, try to take the majority of fluids in the morning and afternoon hours, and limit fluid intake in the hours before bedtime. Second, stop smoking. Nicotine irritates the bladder muscle and causes bladder contractions. Third, eliminate or limit caffeine, alcohol, and carbonated beverages. Aspartame also may aggravate UI symptoms. Women should try eliminating these items one by one to determine which is more troublesome to their symptoms. Finally, if a person is overweight, she should consider weight reduction (Newman & Giovannini, 2002).

Q 7.23   Can fecal constipation aggravate UI?

Yes. Constipation and straining both increase pressure on the bladder. Increase fiber and fluid intake. Increasing one's activity level will enhance bowel motility.

Q 7.24   How does interstitial cystitis fit in with UI?

Interstitial cystitis is manifested by painful, frequent urination accompanied by a sensation of urinary urgency. It is a diagnosis of exclusion and is best managed by a urologist with specialized knowledge of this condition.

Medications and intravesicle therapy (solutions infused into the bladder) are part of a holistic program for ongoing care. Dietary restrictions and stress management techniques are helpful for some individuals, whereas others may require surgery for improvement of symptoms (Gray, Albo, & Huffstutler, 2002).

References

Agency for Health Care Policy and Research. (1996a). *Managing acute and chronic urinary incontinence: Quick reference guide for clinicians* (AHCPR Publication No. 96-0686). Rockville, MD: U.S. Department of Health and Human Services, Public Health Service, Agency for Health Care Policy and Research.

Agency for Health Care Policy and Research. (1996b). *Understanding incontinence: Patient guide* (AHCPR Publication No. 96-0684). Rockville, MD: U.S. Department of Health and Human Services, Public Health Service, Agency for Health Care Policy and Research.

Agency for Health Care Policy and Research. (1996c). *Urinary incontinence in adults: Acute and chronic management* (AHCPR Publication No. 96-0682). Rockville, MD: U.S. Department of Health and Human Services, Public Health Service, Agency for Health Care Policy and Research.

Chiarelli, P.E. (2005). *Women's waterworks: Curing incontinence.* Wallsend, Australia: George Parry.

Chobanian, N. (2002). The business of recycling personal care products. *Quality Care, National Association for Continence, 20*(3), 3.

Doughty, D.B. (Ed.). (1991). *Urinary and fecal incontinence: Nursing management.* St. Louis, MO: Mosby Year Book.

Gray, M. (2002). Are cranberry juice or cranberry products effective in the prevention or management of urinary tract infection? *Journal of Wound, Ostomy and Continence Nursing, 29,* 122–126.

Gray, M., Albo, M., & Huffstutler, S. (2002). Interstitial cystitis: A guide to recognition, evaluation, and management for nurse practitioners. *Journal of Wound, Ostomy and Continence Nursing, 29,* 93–101.

Johnson, V. (2001). How the principles of exercise physiology influence pelvic floor muscle training. *Journal of Wound, Ostomy and Continence Nursing, 28,* 150–154.

Maloney, C. (2002). Estrogen and recurrent UTI in postmenopausal women. *American Journal of Nursing, 102*(8), 44–51.

Newman, D. (2003). Stress urinary incontinence in women. *American Journal of Nursing, 103*(8), 46–56.

Newman, D., & Giovannini, D. (2002). The overactive bladder: A nursing perspective. *American Journal of Nursing, 102*(5), 36–45.

Nygaard, I. (2002). Exercise and urinary incontinence. *Quality Care, National Association for Continence, 20*(2), 1–5.

Weber, A. (2001). Sexual function and urinary incontinence. *Quality Care, National Association for Continence, 19*(4), 1–5.

Resources

Interstitial Cystitis Association: www.ichelp.org
Knowaste Inc.: www.knowaste.com
National Association for Incontinence: www.nafc.org
Wound, Ostomy and Continence Nurses Society: www.wocn.org

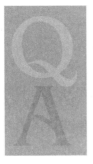

Chapter 8
Fertility Challenges

Lee Ann Ruess, MS, RN, CCRN, CNS, APRN,BC

Background

Q 8.1 What is infertility?

Infertility is defined as the inability to conceive after one year of attempting to achieve pregnancy. For women older than age 35, some say this period should be abbreviated to six months. Approximately 1 in every 6 couples has trouble conceiving. The causes of infertility are mainly male in 30%–40% of cases, mainly female in another 40%, and mixed in 5%–15%. In 15% of cases, a definite cause cannot be identified. These are termed "unexplained infertility" (Centers for Disease Control and Prevention [CDC], 1995).

Q 8.2 What is the difference between infertility and secondary infertility?

"Secondary infertility" applies to situations where women were able to conceive in the past without medical intervention and now seem unable to conceive. Reasons vary greatly but can include mature maternal age, difficulty with prior pregnancy, medical complications, or different partners (Sills, Perloe, Stamm, Kaplan, & Tucker, 2004). Women should consult with their obstetrician/gynecologist (OB/GYN) if they have been trying unsuccessfully for more than a year to conceive or have had a change in their medical condition.

Q 8.3 When should I start seeking medical advice?

Most physicians agree that couples should try to conceive for one year before seeking infertility advice. Women who are 35 or older, who have never conceived before, or who have had recurrent problems with conception should seek advice sooner.

Q __8.4__ **What should I expect when I first discover I have an infertility problem?**

Most OB/GYN healthcare providers will suggest that women track their ovulation schedule. Taking daily temperatures and monitoring their menstrual cycles are early steps. Healthcare providers also will suggest that women use ovulation kits to determine their ovulation cycles. Only after these things are done will they be referred to an infertility specialist for an initial visit and counseling on their options.

Q __8.5__ **There are so many medications. What do they all do?**

Here is an overview of just a few of the many medications women may encounter (Turkoski, Lance, & Bonfiglio, 2004).
- Estrogens: Clomiphene citrate (Clomid®, Aventis, Bridgewater, NJ; Serophene®, Serono, Rockland, MA). Clomiphene is a synthetic drug affecting the estrogen regulation function of the brain. It causes the brain to increase stimulation of the ovaries, thereby increasing estrogen levels and the chance of ovulation. It often is the first line of medications for women who do not ovulate or who ovulate on an irregular basis. Clomiphene can cause a thickening of cervical mucus, making it difficult for sperm to access the egg(s). Treatment usually is artificial insemination.
- Gonadotropins: Gonadotropins are naturally occurring hormones that normally regulate ovarian function. The two kinds of gonadotropins are follicle-stimulating hormone (FSH) and luteinizing hormone (LH). Medications can control both FSH and LH or only FSH. These medications are given intramuscularly either once or twice a day to stimulate follicular growth and estrogen production during the first half of a woman's menstrual cycle. Together, they will increase her chances of producing and releasing an egg(s). Close monitoring by blood work and ultrasound (every two to three days) is required because of how powerful these medications are. The goal is to not overproduce eggs.
- Human chorionic gonadotropin: This medication usually is given after a cycle of gonadotropins to trigger ovulation. It is given by intramuscular injection. Ovulation usually occurs within 36–48 hours of the injection, so this is the best time for intercourse or artificial insemination.

Q __8.6__ **If I do not ovulate regularly, am I infertile?**

Although monthly ovulation typically occurs with a woman's menstrual cycle, some women do not ovulate every month. Some women do not know when they ovulate until they do monthly ovulation tests. Many are still able to get pregnant without intervention by monitoring their cycles and having intercourse before and after ovulation on the months they do ovulate.

8.7 What tests are done to determine infertility?

One of the tests a doctor may suggest is a hysteroscopy. This is minimally invasive outpatient surgery that does not entail the cutting of any normal tissue. It is suitable for the diagnosis and treatment of many conditions, including infertility, painful periods, recurring miscarriages, and menstrual bleeding disorders.

A laparoscopy also is a minimally invasive outpatient surgery technique suitable for diagnosis and correction of infertility, pain, endometriosis, pelvic scarring, and other similar conditions. Laparoscopic surgery requires multiple small punctures into the abdomen to allow visualization of the abdominal and pelvic cavities.

Interventions

8.8 If I use infertility medications, what are my chances of getting pregnant?

Depending on the medication, 5%–30% of women will get pregnant.

8.9 What are the chances of having multiples (twins, triplets, etc.) if I use infertility medications?

Five to ten percent of clomiphene-induced pregnancies result in twins, and less than 1% result in triplets or more. Twenty to thirty percent of gonadotropin-induced pregnancies result in twins. The normal population has a twin rate of 1.2% (CDC, 1995).

8.10 What is the difference between IVF and GIFT?

In vitro fertilization (IVF) is the oldest of the assisted reproductive technique procedures. IVF involves ovulation induction with gonadotropins, office-based vaginal egg retrieval, fertilization with husband/partner/donor sperm in an incubator, and transfer of the resulting embryo(s) through the cervix into the uterus in a simple office procedure. IVF initially was developed for couples with infertility because of tubal blockage, but other causes of infertility also respond to this treatment (Sills, Perloe, et al., 2004).

Gamete intrafallopian transfer (GIFT) involves ovulation induction just as with IVF. The eggs are retrieved during outpatient surgery, mixed with the husband/partner/donor sperm, and returned to the fallopian tube during the same surgery. Because the procedure is done under anesthesia, GIFT offers the option of diagnosing and treating problems such as endometriosis and scar tissue. GIFT requires at least one functioning fallopian tube.

8.11   What is artificial insemination?

Donor (artificial) insemination occurs when the male partner's sperm is obtained by manual ejaculation and then transferred through the woman's cervix in a simple office procedure. The process is used when the male partner has a severely decreased sperm count or if the male has a genetic disorder he does not want to pass to his offspring. It also is used for women without male partners.

Many couples use artificial insemination after taking gonadotropins, which stimulate ovulation, to increase their chances of conception. The chances of conception are likely to be 5%–20% per cycle.

8.12   If I required infertility assistance to get pregnant the first time, will I need it again?

Not necessarily. The menstrual cycle can change throughout a woman's life. The need for subsequent treatment will depend on why she had trouble conceiving in the first place. The patient should consult with her physician.

8.13   What are the risks associated with infertility treatments?

Most studies list cervical cancer, multiple births, and low-birth-weight babies as some of the risks associated with infertility treatments (Sills, Winston, & Palermo, 2004).

8.14   What are some of the common side effects associated with infertility medications?

Side effects include hot flashes, ovarian cysts, ovarian pain, breast tenderness, headache, nervousness, moodiness, irritability, dizziness, nausea/vomiting, fatigue, and visual disturbances. Each woman experiences a different effect from the drugs. Some women experience multiple symptoms, whereas others experience none (Turkoski et al., 2004).

Q 8.15   Now that I understand the physical challenges, what about the emotional ones?

Emotional challenges for women (and men) with infertility issues range from minor to extreme. Couples with infertility problems often feel inadequate as men or women. They may find themselves blaming each other. Women may experience greatly increased hormonal swings while on infertility medications, which adds to the emotional chaos. Couples begin living their lives by "cycle day 10 or 14." To ease the stress, couples should try to focus on their relationship and shared hope of conceiving a baby. The support of caring family members and friends also will help during this time.

Q 8.16   It seems like all I do is wait. Why do treatments take so long?

Everything is based on a woman's menstrual cycle, which is normally 28 days. Certain medications are effective in the early part of the cycle, and others at the end. All the medications and treatments are timed around the production and release of eggs.

Q 8.17   Timing is everything, even when it comes to sex. Is more often better?

Women taking infertility medications often are told when intercourse will increase their chances of conception. But because they cannot precisely predict ovulation, healthcare professionals generally recommend that women have intercourse before and after anticipated times of ovulation. Most physicians will say that "more is better."

References

Centers for Disease Control and Prevention. (1995). *Fertility, family planning, and women's health: Data from NCHS and CDC 1995 national survey of family growth.* Atlanta, GA: Author.

Sills, E.S., Perloe, M., Stamm, L.J., Kaplan, C.R., & Tucker, M.J. (2004). Medical and psychological management of recurrent abortion, history of postneonatal death, ectopic pregnancy and infertility: Successful implementation of IVF for multifactorial reproductive dysfunction. A case report. *Clinical and Experimental Obstetrics and Gynecology, 31,* 143–146.

Sills, E.S., Winston, R.M., & Palermo, G.D. (2004). Shaping the future of research and practice in reproductive endocrinology/infertility. *Journal of Experimental and Clinical Assisted Reproduction, 1*(1), 1.

Turkoski, B.B., Lance, B.R., & Bonfiglio, M.E. (Eds.). (2004). *Drug information handbook for advanced practice nursing* (5th ed.). Hudson, OH: Lexi-Comp.

Resources

American Society for Reproductive Medicine: www.asrm.org
Association of Women's Health, Obstetric and Neonatal Nurses: www.awhonn.org
National Infertility Association: www.resolve.org
Patrizio, P., Tucker, M., & Guelman, V. (Eds.). (2003). *A color atlas for human assisted reproduction: Laboratory and clinical insights.* Philadelphia: Lippincott Williams & Wilkins.

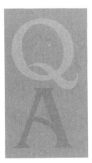

Chapter 9
Depression

Dorothy J. Hall, MS, RN, CNS

Background

Q **9.1** **How do I know whether I have depression or just the blues?**

All people experience the "blues" from time to time, a day or two of feeling "down," when nothing seems right, and motivation is low. One might say, "I'm depressed," but this is quite unlike a true depressive episode. The blues are mild and very short term. Major depression exists at the other end of the spectrum; it can be mild to severe and must be present for at least two weeks for diagnosis. The woman with severe depression has a number of symptoms, is unable to perform at work or school, and has great difficulties with activities of daily living. She may have thoughts of ending her life; she may even have bizarre beliefs or hallucinations. Hospitalization often is necessary. Mild to moderate depression involves less interference with daily functioning and usually can be treated on an outpatient basis.

Between the extremes of the blues and major depression is a condition referred to as dysthymia, or chronic depression. A person who has this form of depression has fewer and perhaps milder symptoms, but the symptoms may continue for many years. This can result in a generally lower level of functioning, limiting a woman's ability to reach her full potential.

Something should be said about bereavement. The signs and reported symptoms associated with mourning the loss of a significant person can look just like depression. However, the "depression" of mourning lacks feelings of worthlessness. About one-third of bereaved people develop a depressive illness one or two months after the loss (Marshall, Atkinson, & the Newcastle Affective Disorders Group, 2001). At that time, a physician may make a diagnosis of depression and begin the patient's treatment.

9.2   Is depression inherited?

Researchers with the National Institute of Mental Health (NIMH, 1999) have found that multiple genes acting together with developmental and environmental factors cause a *vulnerability* to depression and other psychiatric disorders. Other evidence for genetic influence is found in studies of identical twins. If one twin has depression, the other often does also. When several people in a family have depression, the same antidepressant medication often is effective for each of them.

9.3   What causes depression?

Research has shown that depression is caused by an imbalance in brain chemicals called neurotransmitters. The most common of these are serotonin, norepinephrine (or noradrenalin), and dopamine. These chemical substances function to allow the electrical impulses in brain neurons to cross synapses between neurons to reach an effector cell. When the supply of these substances is too low or out of balance, nerve impulses are slowed, resulting in the symptoms of depression. Any kind of stress tends to cause biochemical changes in the brain, thereby increasing the risk of depression in vulnerable individuals.

9.4   I have heard that infections can cause depression. Is that true?

Some medical illnesses such as endocrine disorders and infections are *associated with* depression, possibly causing *symptoms* of depression. As an example, when a patient in a nursing home becomes depressed, a thorough assessment of her condition is in order. In one case, a urinary tract infection was found. Once the infection was treated adequately, the depressive symptoms disappeared.

Some drugs in certain classifications of medications, such as antibiotics, antihypertensives, and steroids, also may cause symptoms of depression, but they do not cause depression.

9.5   Is there a relationship between substance abuse and depression?

Yes, researchers have well established the association between the two. The reason for the relationship, however, is unclear.

One in three depressed people has some form of substance abuse or dependence (National Mental Health Association, 2005). Some people who are depressed choose to "self-medicate" with alcohol in an effort to feel better. This may seem to help in the short run, but because alcohol is a central nervous system depressant, it actually worsens depressive symptoms. Some people may become depressed because of intense guilt feelings about their drinking, the loss of self-esteem, and the loss of important things in their lives (job, relationships, or personal possessions). Depression combined with heavy drinking is very dangerous, with a high risk for suicide. When these two conditions coexist, efforts to treat one without treating the other are ineffective.

9.6 Is depression very prevalent?

Depression occurs in all racial, ethnic, and socioeconomic groups. It is a common illness that affects 20 out of 100 women during their lifetimes (Pavlovich-Danis, 2003). Approximately twice as many women as men are affected by depression (Blehar & Oren, 1999). A number of developmental and environmental factors are thought to play a role in this, such as women's multiple responsibilities at home and at work, single parenting, and caring for aging parents (NIMH, 2000). Other factors include hormonal changes, oppression and victimization of women, and sexual harassment in the workplace. Many women do not get help because the symptoms of depression are mistaken for personal weakness. Symptoms of depression in women often are missed in the primary care setting.

9.7 What are the symptoms of depression?

Feelings of hopelessness, helplessness, and worthlessness are the hallmarks of depression. A woman's reported symptoms represent a change from her previous level of functioning. She may report great sadness, frequent crying spells, a loss of interest in her usual activities, an inability to experience pleasure, and fatigue or loss of energy. Other symptoms may include difficulties with memory and concentration, insomnia or oversleeping, and appetite disturbance with weight loss or weight gain. A person with depression may experience psychomotor agitation or retardation, irritability, negative thoughts, and inappropriate guilt. Anxiety often coexists with depression. The depressed woman most likely feels miserable and may be unable to function on the job or unable to care for the home, cook meals, do laundry, or even maintain personal hygiene. She also may have frequent thoughts of death or suicide, but she may not report these. The healthcare provider should ask whether she has considered ending her life. This will not "push her over the edge." Instead, she very likely will feel relieved that her secret is out.

9.8   How is depression diagnosed?

Unfortunately, no reliable blood test exists that can diagnose depression. The American Psychiatric Association (2000) lists criteria for a diagnosis of depression and other psychiatric illnesses in the *Diagnostic and Statistical Manual of Mental Disorders.* Depression is diagnosed from the particular signs and symptoms and the length of time the symptoms have been present.

9.9   What is SAD, and why is light therapy used?

"SAD" stands for "seasonal affective disorder." This mood disorder is associated with shorter days and decreased exposure to sunlight or lower-intensity sunlight. Some people become depressed at the beginning of winter and remain so until spring. The symptoms differ from those of depression in that people with this condition have an increased appetite and sleep excessively. Approximately 35 million Americans suffer from this disorder ("Seasonal Affective Disorder," 2005). Many people have found that sitting in front of fluorescent, full-spectrum, high-intensity lights for 15–30 minutes daily is beneficial. The lights compensate for the absence of sunshine. Antidepressant medications also have been helpful for this disorder when used during the winter months.

9.10   My friend says I am a "total grouch" for almost two weeks every month. Could I have PMS? Is this the same as depression?

If a woman is moody and irritable and feels depressed or angry prior to her menstrual period, she may have premenstrual syndrome (PMS). A multitude of other mental and physical symptoms have been reported as part of this syndrome. These usually go away with the onset of menses or a few days later. Approximately 3%–5% of reproductive-aged women experience a more severe and debilitating condition called premenstrual dysphoric disorder, which requires treatment (Pavlovich-Danis, 2003). The symptoms may include any of those listed for major depression, as well as food cravings, anxiety, gastrointestinal symptoms, headache, a bloated feeling, and fluid retention. They may be so severe that the woman functions poorly at home, at work, and in interpersonal relationships, in great contrast to her usual level of functioning during the remainder of the month. Treatment usually involves use of an antidepressant medication during the week or two prior to menstruation, adherence to a well-balanced diet with a decrease in salt, regular exercise, stress management, and an increase in daily intake of water. Patients should reduce or eliminate alcohol consumption. Treatment may need to continue until menopause.

9.11   What is postpartum depression?

It is estimated that 30%–75% of new mothers experience the "baby blues" (Seyfried & Marcus, 2003). Symptoms are mild and self-limiting, resolving rapidly without treatment. The new mother with the blues needs someone to listen as she vents her feelings, and she needs reassurance of the transient nature of the condition. Family members need reassurance as well.

Postpartum depression occurs after 10%–15% of deliveries, with its onset occurring within six weeks of childbirth (Seyfried & Marcus, 2003). The new mother experiences many symptoms of major depression, as well as excessive anxiety about the health of the infant. She often has the feeling that she is a failure at motherhood. She may have suicidal tendencies and delusions. This condition frequently is unrecognized, so it is important for the healthcare provider to ask specific questions about the new mother's mood and adjustment to parenthood. Early intervention is important. Healthcare professionals may prescribe antidepressant medications if the mother is not nursing. Sometimes electroconvulsive therapy (ECT) is used.

Postpartum psychosis is severe but rare, occurring in 1–2 women per 1,000 births (Edler, 2002). In this condition, the new mother has several depressive symptoms as well as delusions and possibly hallucinations about the infant. In the latter case, a high risk exists of infanticide or suicide. This is a psychiatric emergency! Protection of the infant and hospitalization of the mother is essential.

9.12   I feel depressed. I am taking medications for hypertension, heart failure, and diabetes. Could any of these be causing my depression?

Both the drug therapies and the conditions themselves are known to be associated with depression. People with diabetes are at greater risk for depression than the general population (NIMH, 2002a), and the same is true for people with heart disease (NIMH, 2002b).

Treatment for depression can help in management of the medical condition. Additionally, medications can be changed or the dosage altered if the side effect of depression becomes apparent. Nonpharmacologic options, such as guided relaxation tapes or other stress management strategies, also can help in controlling symptoms.

9.13   Is suicide very common with depression?

According to NIMH (2003), approximately 1.2 deaths result from suicide per 100 total deaths in the United States, with an estimated 8–25 suicide *attempts* for every completed suicide. The same data show that women attempt suicide about three times as often as men, but four times as many men than women die by suicide. Suicidal *thoughts* are relatively common in people experiencing depression. The individual may feel that her situation is hopeless, that she is worthless and a "burden" to her family. She may believe that her family would be "better off" without her. Death may seem preferable to how she is feeling. It is as though she is wearing blinders and can see no other option.

9.14   How should I approach someone who is talking about suicide?

Respond to her with concern, and do not minimize her statements or judge her. She may be crying out for help. Any person who talks about suicide should be taken seriously. Most suicidal people do not want to "die and be dead forever" but want to "stop living the way I am living." Almost everyone who is thinking about suicide gives some sort of clue. The person may make direct statements such as "I wish I were dead" or "I'm going to kill myself," or indirect statements such as "I hate my life; I hate everything" or "my family would be better off without me." She may start giving away treasured possessions. Any of these statements or actions should be taken seriously. Arrange for her to see her healthcare provider, and enlist the assistance of family members as necessary. If she has a plan for when and how she will end her life or has access to the chosen method, *do not leave her alone.* Get help immediately! An emergency room assessment is appropriate. Consider the questions used by this author in assessment of suicide risk.

• Are there thoughts of suicide as a solution to current problems?
• Have there been previous suicide attempts? Previous attempts or history of suicide in the family increases the risk.
• Has the person made a plan? If the plan is specific, the risk is higher.

- Has the person chosen a method?
- How lethal is the method chosen? Gunshots or hanging are more lethal than medication overdose.
- Does the person have access to the method chosen? If not, it would take more time to act. If so, the situation is urgent. If prescription bottles are lined up on the table or a gun is on the sofa next to the person or anywhere in the house, time is critical. Call 911 or the local emergency service and stay with the person until help arrives.

Treatment

9.15 How is depression treated?

Medication, psychotherapy, or a combination of both can treat depression. Approximately 80% of patients will improve with adequate antidepressant therapy (NIMH, 1999) for the proper length of time. The results are the same for psychotherapy.

9.16 What medications are best for treating depression?

None of the many antidepressant medications is considered "best." All are effective, but some may be better for certain kinds of depression, such as depression associated with anxiety. All antidepressants increase the neuronal transmission of serotonin, norepinephrine, and/or dopamine. Some mild improvement in symptoms, particularly sleep and appetite, may be seen in two weeks. However, it may take 6–12 weeks after the therapeutic dosage of medication has been reached for full benefit to be seen.

For many years, **tricyclic antidepressants**, named for their chemical structure, were the only treatments for depression other than ECT. Today, drugs in this classification are used infrequently because newer drugs have fewer side effects, are better tolerated, and are safer if taken in overdose. The prototype drug in this category is amitriptyline.

Very often, one of the **selective serotonin reuptake inhibitors** (SSRIs) is the first choice in treating newly diagnosed depression. These often are effective for anxiety as well as depression. Examples in this category are fluoxetine, paroxetine, and sertraline. Other very closely related drugs may be used as well.

Monoamine oxidase inhibitors (MAOIs) are used very rarely at this time. They were used in the past if several medications from the tricyclic category were ineffective. Severe dietary restrictions are necessary for patients taking an MAOI. Failure to avoid foods and medicines containing tyramine can precipitate a potentially fatal hypertensive crisis in a person taking an MAOI. There must be a two-week delay between stopping other antidepressants and starting MAOIs and vice versa to prevent serious and potentially fatal reactions.

9.17   How do antidepressant medications work?

The function of antidepressant medication is to facilitate the transfer of electric nerve impulses across the synapse. More than two dozen antidepressant medications exist, with more than six mechanisms of action (Stahl, 1997). By one or more of these mechanisms, neurotransmitters are aided in effective transfer of the nerve impulse from one neuron to the next and the next. This process allows the nerve impulse to continue to its destination, resulting in improvement of symptoms.

9.18   What are the side effects of antidepressant medication?

Tricyclic antidepressants such as amitriptyline have the potential for causing serious side effects such as cardiac dysrhythmias, orthostatic hypotension, paralytic ileus, and excessive sedation. These could be especially dangerous for older adults or those who work around dangerous machinery. Because of the potential for cardiac dysrhythmias, medications in this category usually are fatal if an overdose is taken. Other side effects include dry mouth, constipation, difficulty urinating, and worsening of glaucoma.

SSRIs and other related antidepressant medications have annoying side effects that usually go away during treatment. Some people will experience nausea and/or headaches during the early phase of treatment, and they may be advised to take the medication after a meal. These symptoms usually wear off as the body gets accustomed to the medication. Most drugs in this category cause increased appetite with potential weight gain, decreased libido, and possibly anorgasmia. SSRIs and related antidepressants usually are not lethal if the patient takes an overdose.

As with all medications, particular caution is necessary with regard to drug interactions. Several of the newer antidepressants affect liver metabolism of medications given for other conditions. This can result in decreased blood concentration and poor benefit from the other medications or increased blood concentration of the other medications along with toxicity.

Q 9.19   Can I stop the medication as soon as I feel better?

No. The patient will continue on antidepressants for six months to one year after the depression has lifted and she is functioning well again. The patient and her healthcare provider together decide the appropriate time to attempt stopping the medication. The decision depends on the level and length of improvement and is made only if all else is stable in the patient's life. An attempt at reduction of dosage is *not* made if a person has just lost a job or is starting a new one, is graduating, is getting married or divorced, or is going through some other major, life-changing event. When the time is right, the medication is reduced gradually. Both physician and patient then watch for signs of relapse.

Q 9.20   Does a person ever have to continue medication for life?

Some patients treated for depression with antidepressant medications and psychotherapy can stop the medication after an appropriate length of time and will not have a recurrence. Approximately 70% experience relapse, and nearly half of these have a chronic depression that requires lifelong treatment (Lazowick, 1997).

Q 9.21   Are "shock treatments" still used to treat depression?

ECT is a very effective treatment for depression, but stigmas remain from the days when patients were not anesthetized and had broken bones from the grand mal seizures. Today, healthcare providers give ECT under general anesthesia, along with muscle relaxants, and use lower voltages. For this reason, very little body movement occurs, perhaps just a twitch in the big toe. The patient usually awakens within 15 minutes and may briefly experience confusion. Short-term memory loss is common and worsens during the series of treatments but resolves a few weeks after treatments end (Rother, 2003). Patients may receive ECT if they have tried several different antidepressants at an appropriate dose for an appropriate length of time and have had minimal to no benefit. It also may be used when the situation is urgent to gain rapid relief from symptoms, and it may be safer than medications for a woman who is pregnant (Rother). Patients receive a series of treatments followed by less-frequent maintenance therapy. Improvement from ECT is dramatic in 80%–90% of people with severe depression (NIMH, 1999).

Q 9.22   Once a depressed and suicidal person begins medication, can I stop worrying that she might attempt suicide?

No. She needs to be watched even more closely then. During the first few days and weeks of treatment, the risk of a suicide attempt increases. Sleep and energy often improve prior to any improvement in mood and thought. The person then may have enough energy to follow through with her suicide plan. Remember that it can take up to eight weeks for full benefit from antidepressants to be seen. Encourage the person to be patient with herself and to avoid comparing symptoms day to day. She likely will feel more hopeful if she looks at "this week compared to last week."

Q 9.23   I heard that many hospitalized patients are depressed. Is this because they are overly worried about their illness, surgery, or recovery?

Naturally, women needing hospitalization for illness and/or surgery are stressed, and they may be very anxious and even tearful. This is not necessarily depression. However, some women may have depression along with the medical condition for which they are hospitalized. That is the case for an estimated 10%–14% of hospitalized patients (National Mental Health Association, 2005). Depression in hospitalized patients may be missed because caregivers assume the patient is simply upset about the illness, or the caregiver is not aware of the presentation of depression. Identification of depression and arranging treatment are important.

Q 9.24   What can you tell me about manic depression?

Manic depression is now called "bipolar disorder." This name is based on the characteristic fluctuations between severe depression and an irritable or very elevated mood. During the manic phase with the elevated and/or irritable mood, the patient also may have an inflated self-image, excess energy, rapid and loud speech, little need for sleep, and a tendency toward impulsive actions such as overspending and sexual promiscuity (Marken, 1997). Several variations of bipolar disorder exist. Healthcare providers do not treat patients with this disorder with antidepressant medication, as these drugs can precipitate a manic episode. Patients have received treatment with lithium carbonate for many years. Anticonvulsant medications now are being used frequently. The U.S. Food and Drug Administration has approved olanzapine (Zyprexa®, Eli Lilly, Indianapolis, IN), an antipsychotic, for bipolar disorder, although it can cause serious side effects and must be used with caution (*Olanzapine*, 2005; *Zyprexa*, 2004).

Q 9.25   How does psychotherapy help a depressed person?

A psychiatric nurse with an advanced degree or a master's-prepared social worker, counselor, or psychologist can provide therapy for depressed patients. The psychotherapist guides the patient to recognize and use her available coping skills for getting through the difficult early days of treatment. These might include calling a friend, listening to music, taking a walk, or calling upon her Higher Power. One idea is to make a "coping menu," listing activities and resources from which a person can choose. The phone number of the community's emergency mental health center always should be included, along with 911 in case the person should feel overtly suicidal.

During psychotherapy, the healthcare professional should remind the person of the time required for medications to work and for healing to take place. She is reminded of the need to take one day or one hour at a time. Other strategies, such as exercise, are very important for the depressed woman as well. Often the plan is to start slowly and build exercise tolerance. For example, the woman may be asked to begin by walking from her house to the house next door twice a day for a week, then to gradually increase the distance walked.

It also is very important to teach a depressed person to recognize how thoughts, and not events themselves, create painful emotions. People can interpret events in different ways, some of which can be very negative. For example, a depressed person may perceive that a friend does not come to visit because "she doesn't like me any more," when the reality is that the friend has been out of town all week. It takes time to learn these skills of managing thoughts and feelings, and the process of reviewing events may need to be repeated many times in therapy.

Q 9.26   How can I help my friend who appears to be depressed?

People should listen to a friend who seems depressed. Let her talk about her concern, worry, sorrow, and other feelings. Do not minimize her feelings or give advice. Just listen and make sure she knows that others hear her and care about her. Do not be afraid to ask if she is feeling depressed. Suggest that she consider talking to her healthcare provider about her feelings, and remind her that depression is quite treatable. Ask whether she has thoughts of harming herself or ending her life. This will not lead her to attempt suicide. She may be relieved that someone cared enough to ask. Help her make arrangements to get help. If she has a *plan* for suicide, get help immediately. This may include getting her family involved or taking her to the local emergency room for assessment. Then be available as a friend and support person during the difficult road back to health.

References

American Psychiatric Association. (2000). *Diagnostic and statistical manual of mental disorders* (4th ed., text rev.). Washington, DC: Author.

Blehar, M., & Oren, D. (1999). Gender differences in depression. *Medscape General Medicine, 1*(2). Retrieved October 14, 2005, from http://www.medscape.com/viewarticle/408844

Edler, C.R. (2002). Beyond the baby blues: Postpartum depression. *Nursing Spectrum (Midwest), 3*(10), 24–29.

Lazowick, A.L. (1997). Managing patients with depression. *Drug Topics Supplement, 141,* 40s–43s.

Marken, P.A. (1997). Current treatment issues in bipolar disorder. *Drug Topics Supplement, 141,* 18s–22s.

Marshall, P.J., Atkinson, C., & the Newcastle Affective Disorders Group. (2001, May). *Grief, bereavement and depression.* Retrieved October 14, 2005, from http://community.netdoktor.com/ccs/uk/depression/coping/social/article.jsp?articleIdent=uk.depression.coping.social.uk_depression_article_1708

National Institute of Mental Health. (1999). *Depression research at the National Institute of Mental Health.* Retrieved July 26, 2005, from http://www.nimh.nih.gov/publicat/depresfact.cfm

National Institute of Mental Health. (2000). *Depression: What every woman should know.* Retrieved July 25, 2005, from http://www.nimh.nih.gov/publicat/depwomenknows.cfm

National Institute of Mental Health. (2002a). *Depression and diabetes.* Retrieved July 26, 2005, from http://www.nimh.nih.gov/publicat/depdiabetes.cfm

National Institute of Mental Health. (2002b). *Depression and heart disease.* Retrieved June 14, 2005, from http://www.nimh.nih.gov/publicat/depheart.cfm

National Institute of Mental Health. (2003, April). *In harm's way: Suicide in America.* Retrieved July 15, 2005, from http://www.nimh.nih.gov/publicat/harmaway.cfm

National Mental Health Association. (2005). *Co-occurrence of depression with medical, psychiatric, and substance abuse disorders.* Retrieved July 28, 2005, from http://www.nmha.org/infoctr/factsheets/28.cfm

Olanzapine. (2005, January). Retrieved September 7, 2005, from http://www.nlm.nih.gov/medlineplus/druginfo/medmaster/a601213.html

Pavlovich-Danis, S.J. (2003, March). Cyclic upheaval—premenstrual syndrome and premenstrual dysphoric disorder. *Nursing Spectrum (Midwest), 4*(3), 26–30.

Rother, L.F. (2003). Electroconvulsive therapy sheds its shocking image. *Nursing, 33*(3), 48–49.

Seasonal affective disorder: Sunbox offers treatment option for seasonal affective disorder sufferers. (2005, January 10). *Health and Medicine Week,* p. 1232.

Seyfried, L.S., & Marcus, S.M. (2003). Postpartum mood disorders. *International Review of Psychiatry, 15,* 231–242.

Stahl, S.M. (1997). *Psychopharmacology of antidepressants.* London: Martin Dunitz.

Zyprexa. (2004, April). Retrieved September 7, 2005, from http://www.psycheducation. org/depression/meds/olanzapine.htm

Resources

Golant, M., & Golant, S.K. (1996). *What to do when someone you love is depressed.* New York: Henry Holt.

National Institute of Mental Health: www.nimh.nih.gov

National Mental Health Association: www.nmha.org

Chapter 10
Sexually Transmitted Infections

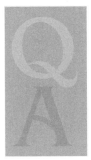

Janet Akers, MSN, RN, CEN

Background

Q 10.1 What is a sexually transmitted infection (STI)?

STIs are illnesses that are spread by having sex with someone who is infected with a causative organism. People can get an STI from sexual activity that involves the mouth, anus, vagina, or penis. STIs previously were called sexually transmitted diseases or venereal diseases. Healthcare professionals have identified more than 20 diseases that are transmitted through sexual activity, with an associated cost in the United States estimated to be more than $10 billion per year (National Institute of Allergy and Infectious Diseases [NIAID], 2003b).

Q 10.2 How common are STIs?

Approximately 13 million Americans will contract an STI each year; more than half of them are younger than age 25 (NIAID, 2003b). The rate actually may be higher because many infections are asymptomatic, and people may not realize they have one until the infection is severe.

Q 10.3 Can STIs be cured?

STIs are distinguished by viral, bacterial, protozoan, and other causative organisms. Bacterial STIs include gonorrhea, chlamydia, bacterial vaginosis, and syphilis. Protozoan STIs include trichomoniasis; others include pubic lice and scabies. These can be "cured" with medications.

Viral STIs *cannot* be cured. These include HIV, hepatitis B (HBV), herpes, and human papillomavirus (HPV). The symptoms can be treated, but the virus remains and can be transmitted to a sexual partner.

Q 10.4   What are the risk factors for STIs?

Some risk factors include multiple sexual partners, use of alcohol and drugs, failure to use condoms or latex barriers or incorrect use of the barriers, sexual relations with partners who have an STI, lack of knowledge about STIs, being female, and being younger than age 25. Another risk factor is incomplete treatment. The infected person must seek treatment for the infection and must take all medication as prescribed. If the partner needs medication, then he or she should be tested and get a prescription. If partners have been diagnosed with an STI, they must not share medications. If medications are shared, then neither partner gets a complete dose. The STI can continue, and both will become infected again.

Q 10.5   Why is being female a particular concern regarding STIs?

Symptoms tend to not be apparent in women with STIs. Therefore, they may not seek treatment until a problem has become advanced. This can result in damage to the uterus and/or fallopian tubes, leading to infertility or an ectopic pregnancy. Also, a connection exists between STIs and cervical cancer (NIAID, 2003b).

Q 10.6   What are some myths about STIs?

Some of the more common myths involve thinking that certain behaviors before or after sex will prevent an STI. Some people believe that douching, urinating, using birth control pills, and washing the genitals after sex are effective protection. None of these will prevent STIs, and they may cause irritation that increases a person's risk of getting an STI. Another myth is that condoms or latex barriers protect against all STIs. Barriers protect against many STIs, but skin-to-skin contact still occurs above the end of the condom. Some infections can be passed from this skin-to-skin contact, even with the use of a condom.

Another myth is that if a person cannot see symptoms, then the partner does not have an STI. Many people have STIs and do not have symptoms. Both partners need to receive regular checkups and STI screening if they are sexually active. Individuals should take care of themselves and insist on protection and safer sex practices. A person should have sex only when he or she wants to and when it is safe. Only an individual can be sure of his or her own monogamy.

Q 10.7   What can I do to prevent getting an STI?

Abstaining from sex is the most effective way to prevent getting an STI. If people choose to engage in sexual relations, they can do things to reduce their risk of getting an STI. People can use a latex condom or barrier every time they have sex. If using a lubricant, they should make sure it is water based. Oil-based lubricants destroy condoms and latex barriers. One can practice monogamy by having only one sexual partner and requiring that the partner not have sex with anyone else. People should choose their sexual partners with care and should not have sex with someone who they think has an STI. Also, people should get checked for STIs so they do not give an STI to someone else. Refrain from using drugs or alcohol before having sex. A person who is drunk or high may take risks that he or she would not usually take or may forget to use a condom. People should learn the signs and symptoms of STIs and look for them in themselves and their partner. Leave the lights on when starting a sexual activity. If people cannot see, they cannot look for symptoms of an STI. If people cannot see or the partner will not let him or her look, they should not have sex.

Talk with a potential sex partner before having sex. Ask about his or her sexual history. Ask about the number of partners and whether the potential partner has ever been told he or she has an STI, including HBV or hepatitis C (HCV) or HIV/AIDS. Ask about high-risk behaviors that may increase the risk for blood diseases such as hepatitis or HIV. High-risk behaviors include IV drug use, anal sex, homosexual sex, sex with a prostitute, sex with other partners who have high-risk behaviors, and exchanges of sex for money or drugs. Ask potential sex partners to be tested for HIV and other STIs. Both partners should use condoms for all sex until they each have not had sex with another person for six months, and then get tested again.

All sexually active people should get routine health exams and screening for STIs. For women, this includes Pap smears. IV drug users should not share needles or syringes. Do not share instruments for ear piercing, tattooing, or hair removal, as well as toothbrushes or razors. If not already vaccinated, get the vaccination for hepatitis A (HAV) and HBV. Avoid kissing or having oral sex with a partner who has open sores in his or her mouth.

Avoid having sex during menstruation. Women are more susceptible to becoming infected with HIV during this time. Women should

Q 10.8   Women's Health: A Resource Guide for Nurses

avoid douching, as this activity removes some of the normal protective bacteria in the vagina.

Remember that anyone can have an STI, may not have symptoms, and may not be aware of having an infection. Get tested, use condoms or barriers until both partners are tested, and remain monogamous.

Q 10.8   If I think I have an STI, where can I go to get help?

Many counties have public health clinics that offer testing and treatment for free or at minimal cost. People can contact the American Social Health Association at 800-227-8922 for information on local clinics and physicians who provide treatment for people with STIs. Individuals enrolled in a university that has a health service may be able to seek assistance there. Another option would be an urgent care center.

Types of Sexually Transmitted Infections

Q 10.9   What is chlamydia?

Chlamydia is the number-one bacterial STI in the United States today, affecting more than three million people. It is known as the silent epidemic because most people with the infection have no symptoms.

Complications from chlamydia can include pelvic inflammatory disease (PID), damage to the fallopian tubes that could result in infertility or ectopic pregnancy, chronic pelvic pain from adhesions (scar tissue), testicular infections, eye infections in adults and newborns, pneumonia in the newborn, and sexually acquired reactive arthritis (Reiter syndrome), which is most commonly seen in men (NIAID, 2004a). Treatment is an oral antibiotic. All partners should be treated at the same time to avoid passing the infection back and forth. Pregnant women should be tested and treated to prevent infections in the newborn during passage through the birth canal. Patients must finish the full course of antibiotics, even if the symptoms stop. If not, the infection may remain.

Q 10.10   What is herpes?

Herpes is a chronic viral infection. Major symptoms are sores or blisters in the genital area. The infection is caused by the herpes simplex virus. Each year, approximately 500,000 new people become infected (NIAID, 2003b).

Early symptoms may feel like a burning sensation in the genitals, lower back pain, pain with urinating, and flu-like symptoms. After a few days, small red bumps may appear in the genital area. These bumps can develop into painful blisters that crust over, form a scab, and then heal within two to three weeks. Other symptoms may be itching, burning, or tingling in the genital area, mouth, legs, or buttocks; fever; or swollen lymph nodes.

Once the virus has been transmitted and the first outbreak has occurred, the virus becomes dormant. Outbreaks occur from time to time when the virus travels from the nerves to the skin and causes blisters and sores. The virus remains in the body for life, and a person has an average of four to five outbreaks a year. Over time, the recurrences lessen in severity and frequency. Outbreaks can be triggered by stress, excessive exposure to the sun, physical injury, fatigue, illness, surgery, vigorous sex, diet, and hormone changes with monthly menses (NIAID, 2003a). Each person is different, and the pattern of outbreaks varies greatly. Recent research suggests that reduction in chronic stress can minimize secondary outbreaks of the virus (Kohl, 2003).

Complications also can include transmission to a baby if the mother acquires herpes during pregnancy. Herpes during pregnancy has been associated with miscarriage, stillbirth, prematurity, severe fetal brain injury, and blindness in the baby. However, many women with herpes have healthy babies. A baby will be delivered by cesarean section if active lesions are present when the expectant mother goes into labor. It is very important that women discuss their illness with their primary healthcare provider and/or their obstetrician.

Patients receive antiviral medications for treatment. Although the drugs can control symptoms, they do not eradicate the virus from the body. In addition to medications, comfort measures such as warm baths and mild analgesics may be helpful. Keep the sores clean and dry. Use a hair dryer on low setting to dry the sores—this may be more comfortable than rubbing with a towel. Wash hands frequently to avoid transmitting the virus. Avoid sexual activity any time a lesion is present. Eating a good diet, getting enough rest, and getting regular exercise may reduce the number and severity of outbreaks.

Q 10.11 What is gonorrhea?

The bacterium *Neisseria gonorrhoeae* causes gonorrhea. This infection can lead to complications such as PID. The bacteria grow in the warm, moist areas of the reproductive tract such as the cervix, uterus, and fallopian tubes. Transmission is from vaginal cervical secretions and semen and from mother to newborn during childbirth. No symptoms may exist. If present, symptoms may occur within 2–10 days and include yellowish vaginal discharge and burning or pain with urination. Women also may have lower back pain, abdominal pain, pain with intercourse, nausea, fever, and bleeding between monthly periods (Schaffer, 2004).

Treatment with a single dose of an antibiotic can cure the infection. Frequently, gonorrhea and chlamydia occur together, so combined treatment with several drugs may be used (NIAID, 2004b).

Q 10.12   What is HPV?

HPV is the number-one viral STI in the United States today. HPV is actually a group of more than 100 different types of viruses. Approximately 30 of these types are spread through sexual contact, and several are known to cause cancer. It is estimated that 20 million Americans are infected, and 5.5 million new cases are diagnosed each year in the United States (Parch, 2003). Symptoms can range from nothing to soft, pink, cauliflower-shaped warts to hard, smooth, gray warts. The warts are not easily visible in women, as they may be in the vagina or anus or on the cervix. The warts may appear between three weeks and six months after having sex with a partner who is infected with HPV. Transfer of the virus is from skin-to-skin contact. If left untreated, the warts may disappear, but the virus remains, and warts may reappear.

Diagnosis is made by a physical examination of the skin or Pap smear of the cervix to detect the warts. Studies have shown that HPV is the major cause of cervical cancer (National Cancer Institute, 2003). No cure exists. Treatment focuses on removal of the warts for comfort and appearance. Removal of warts can be done by cryotherapy or application of a mild acid. In severe cases, laser surgery may be needed. The three procedures can be done in a clinic or doctor's office with a local anesthetic.

During pregnancy, healthcare providers will delay treatment until after delivery unless the warts are blocking the birth canal. If this occurs, they usually will deliver the baby by a cesarean section. Risk of transmission of the virus to the baby is very low (Parch, 2003).

Patients can best prevent HPV by avoiding sex with a partner who is infected. Condoms may provide some protection if they cover the area of infection. Women need to have regular Pap smears; those who have been diagnosed with cervical warts should have Pap smears every six months to check for changes in cervical cells.

10.13   What is syphilis?

The bacterium *Treponema pallidum* causes syphilis. Once very common, syphilis now is one of the least common STIs in the United States. Syphilis is spread through direct contact with a lesion or through transplacental infection of the fetus. It cannot be spread by toilet seats, doorknobs, pools, hot tubs, bathtubs, or sharing clothing or eating utensils. It is spread by having sex with an infected partner when chancres (painless ulcerated lesions, pronounced "shankers") or rash are present.

A unique feature of this STI is that it has four stages (Bankowski & Bankowski, 2003).
- Stage one: Known as primary syphilis, this can be mistaken for other conditions. In this stage, people can develop one or more chancre sores. They can occur on the genitals or around the mouth. They appear 10–90 days after a person is infected and heal in about six weeks. During this stage, people are highly contagious, but the infection can be treated easily with an antibiotic.
- Stage two: Known as the secondary stage, this may last one to three months and starts an average of six months after a person becomes infected. Infected people may develop a rash on the palms of their hands or the soles of their feet. Moist warts may be present in the groin, in addition to white patches on the inside of the mouth, sore throat, swollen lymph nodes, fever, weight loss, patchy hair loss of the eyebrows and lashes, headaches, irritability, unequal reflexes, and irregular pupils. This stage will resolve by itself.
- Stage three: This is known as latent syphilis. The infection lies dormant without causing symptoms and can last for years. The average is 2–20 years and has lasted as long as 46 years.
- Stage four: Called "tertiary syphilis," this occurs if the infection is not treated. The hallmarks of this stage are severe problems with the heart (cardiovascular syphilis), brain, and nerves (neurosyphilis). A person may become blind, impotent, or demented or even

may die without treatment. The damage at this stage may be irreversible.

Healthcare providers diagnose syphilis easily with a blood test and treat it with antibiotics. The amount and type depends on what stage of the disease an individual is determined to have. To prevent the spread of the STI, patients should not have sex until all sores have healed completely. All partners must be tested and treated as appropriate. Antibiotics are effective in any stage. However, antibiotics cannot reverse the damage done by the complications of tertiary syphilis. They only can prevent further complications from developing.

If a woman is pregnant and has syphilis, the bacteria cross the placenta and can infect the baby at any time of the pregnancy. Once infected, the baby can be stillborn or die shortly after birth. The baby may be born without symptoms and then develop them in a few weeks. A baby born with congenital syphilis but not treated may become developmentally delayed, have seizures, or die.

Q 10.14   What is HIV/AIDS?

Acquired immune deficiency syndrome (AIDS) was first reported in the United States in 1981. It is caused by the human immunodeficiency virus (HIV). The virus destroys the body's ability to fight off infections and cancers. Rates of infection and death are particularly high among women of color, to a large extent because of limited access to appropriate and timely health care. Transmission is through sexual activity, by sharing needles used to inject drugs intravenously, or during pregnancy, delivery, or breast-feeding. The transmission of HIV is increased in the presence of certain other STIs (Smith & Schaffer, 2004).

No symptoms occur from HIV itself. Nonspecific symptoms may be present that are similar to influenza or infection. The transition from HIV to late-stage disease, or AIDS, occurs as the number of marker cells (CD4+) decline and significant opportunistic infections set in.

Symptoms of AIDS usually are the same as those for the opportunistic infection or cancer. They may include fever, chills, sweats, fatigue, weight loss, muscle and joint pain, sore throat, swollen lymph nodes, diarrhea, yeast infections, and skin sores. Frequently a person with AIDS develops Kaposi sarcoma, *Pneumocystis carinii* pneumonia, tuberculosis, meningitis, or herpes infections. The symptoms can last for weeks or months and do not go away without treatment.

Healthcare providers make a diagnosis from blood, urine, or oral testing for the antibodies to the virus. It may take three to six months for enough antibodies to be detected. If people think they have been exposed or want to know whether they have HIV, they should discuss testing with a healthcare provider, get the testing, and then be retested in six months to confirm the results of the first test if it was negative.

All sex partners and anyone with whom a person has shared needles and syringes need to be told that they may have been exposed to the virus. They all should be tested for HIV.

No cure or vaccine exists for HIV or AIDS. Although once considered fatal, healthcare professionals now consider HIV to be a treatable chronic infection. Medications and combinations of medications can control symptoms and expand longevity. A key to effective treatment is to commit to taking a complicated regimented schedule of medicines exactly as prescribed and consistently. Patients must not miss a dose or stop taking the medications.

HIV and AIDS have significant psychosocial implications, as well. The condition may cause disruption in normal lifestyle, employment, and relationships. Insurance coverage and access to needed health care may become challenging. As the condition progresses, fear of acquiring an opportunistic infection becomes very real, and patients must take stringent precautions to safeguard their health. Families of people with HIV/AIDS experience dramatic effects, as does the person with the diagnosis. A woman who has a spouse or significant other with the condition also will need psychosocial support.

10.15 What is hepatitis?

Hepatitis is inflammation of the liver because of viral infection, with the type of hepatitis identified by alphabet letters. Hepatitis A, B, and C are the most well known of the hepatitis viruses. HAV is the most common, followed by HBV, and then HCV. HAV is rarely chronic but can cause a life-threatening infection. HBV and HCV can be acute or chronic as well as life threatening. The viruses can cause liver scarring, liver failure, and cancer.

HAV most frequently is found in the stool. Fecal-oral contamination is the usual transmission route. Although usually associated with food workers or daycare providers when hand washing is not done or is done incorrectly, HAV also can be transmitted if partners engage in anal sex. The HAV vaccine is effective.

HBV is the hepatitis virus usually associated with STIs. Transmission is through blood and body fluids. The vaccine is effective and has resulted in a significant decline in the number of HBV cases in the United States since 1982; however, the vaccine should not be given to those allergic to yeast (Centers for Disease Control and Prevention, 2005).

HCV usually is associated with blood transfusions and with the sharing of contaminated needles and syringes. No vaccine exists for HCV.

Symptoms of acute hepatitis infection may include jaundice, light-colored stool, unexplained fatigue that lasts for months, fever, nausea, vomiting, loss of appetite, and abdominal pain. It may take one to six months after exposure for the symptoms to appear. Physicians make a diagnosis after a physical exam and blood tests and may include liver biopsies.

Treatment is aimed at the symptoms and reduction of the amount of virus present in the liver. Rest and diet changes are important treatments. Pregnant women can spread the virus to the baby during birth. Newborns infected with HBV can develop long-term liver problems. All newborns should receive vaccination at birth and in the first year of life. No cures exist for HAV, HBV, or HCV.

If a person has a chronic form of hepatitis, he or she should not donate blood, plasma, organs, sperm, or tissue. Infected people also should avoid alcoholic beverages and should not take supplements or herbs unless their physician is aware. Some herbal remedies can cause the liver damage to become worse.

10.16   Is a vaginal infection an STI?

A vaginal infection may be symptomatic of an STI or may occur because of other organisms, foreign bodies, or irritants. Vaginal discharge and itching are the most common symptoms. Treatment depends on the causative agent. Testing may be done to rule out a causative or related STI.

Prevention/Detection

Q 10.17   Should I get tested routinely for STIs if I am sexually active?

Testing to determine STI status for both an individual and his or her new partner is recommended when starting a new sexual relationship. If a person has multiple partners, routine testing is even more important. People should discuss with their healthcare provider how often they should be screened for STIs. The more partners a person has, the more frequently screening should be done. If both partners have tested negative for STIs and are committed to having sexual relations only with each other, then routine testing specifically for STIs is not necessary. However, usual health screenings, including pelvic examinations and Pap smears, will include discussions with their healthcare provider about their sexual health.

Q 10.18   What things should I consider before having sex with a new partner?

Before starting a sexual relationship, people should ask themselves and the new partner the following questions.
- Why am I thinking about having sex with this partner? Do I want to, or is it because he or she is pressuring me to have sex?
- How many sexual partners has the new person had, and how many have I had?
- Are we both willing to be monogamous with each other?
- Are we both willing to use condoms or latex barriers?
- Are we both willing to be tested for STIs, including HIV/AIDS?
- Has the new partner ever had an STI, or does he or she have one now?
- Do I have an STI? Am I willing to tell the new partner?
- Does my new partner want me to engage in anal sex?
- Do I know the signs and symptoms of STIs?
- Are we both willing to not use drugs and alcohol before having sex?

Q 10.19   How can I tell if my sex partner has an STI?

Sometimes no symptoms are present, and without testing, an individual may not know if his or her partner has an STI. However, if symptoms are present, they may include one or more of the following: bumps, sores, blisters, or warts near the mouth, anus, penis, or vagina; swelling or redness near the penis or vagina; painful urination; rapid or constant weight loss, loose stools, and night sweats; fever, chills, aches, and pains; discharge from the penis or vagina; painful sex or pain in the testicles; severe itching near the penis or vagina or in the genital area; and yellowish skin or eye color.

Q 10.20   I was just diagnosed with an STI. Should my sex partner get tested?

Yes. Not only should the partner get tested, but the partner should be treated as well. Without both people getting treated, the STI can continue to be passed back and forth. While a person has an STI, he or she should not have sex. If the partner refuses to be tested and/or treated, the individual should not have sex with the partner.

Q 10.21   How do I tell my partner I have an STI?

People can communicate to a partner that they have an STI in several ways. The direct approach may be effective. People with an STI should talk directly to their partner about the STI and the partner's need for testing and treatment. They should be prepared that they or the partner could become angry or hurt. They need to educate themselves and the partner about the STI. Remember, some STIs may be present for months or years without symptoms, and having one does not always mean someone had sex with another person outside the relationship. Encourage the partner to seek medical treatment. Counseling with a healthcare provider may help both partners to understand how the STI was transmitted.

An indirect approach can be used to tell a casual partner, such as a note left for the partner with information that he or she may have been exposed to an STI and should be tested and treated as soon as possible. The note can include a phone number for a health clinic that will provide confidential testing. Some health department clinics have preprinted forms with information about STIs and where to get tested and treated.

Q 10.22   Can I get an STI from a sex toy?

If the sex toy is used in the vagina, anus, or mouth of a person who has an STI present in any of those areas, the toy can become contaminated. If the sex toy is then inserted into the mouth, anus, or vagina of the partner, the STI can be transferred. All sex toys should be washed with soap and water after each use. If unsure whether a sexual partner has an STI, a condom or latex barrier could be used on the toy. Do not insert the toy into one opening and then into another opening without cleaning it or changing the barrier.

References

Bankowski, S.B., & Bankowski, B. (2003). The silent STD epidemic: An overview. In L. Gerdes (Ed.), *Sexually transmitted diseases* (pp. 19–25). San Diego, CA: Greenhaven Press.

Centers for Disease Control and Prevention. (2005, August). *Viral hepatitis B fact sheet*. Retrieved September 9, 2005, from http://www.cdc.gov/ncidod/diseases/hepatitis/b/fact.htm

Kohl, M. (2003). Stress reduction may control the recurrence of genital herpes. In L. Gerdes (Ed.), *Sexually transmitted diseases* (pp. 119–120). San Diego, CA: Greenhaven Press.

National Cancer Institute. (2003). The relationship between human papillomaviruses and cancer. In L. Gerdes (Ed.), *Sexually transmitted diseases* (pp. 46–49). San Diego, CA: Greenhaven Press.

National Institute of Allergy and Infectious Diseases. (2003a, September). *Genital herpes*. Retrieved September 8, 2005, from http://www.niaid.nih.gov/factsheets/stdherp.htm

National Institute of Allergy and Infectious Diseases. (2003b, November). *An introduction to sexually transmitted infections*. Retrieved September 8, 2005, from http://www.niaid.nih.gov/publications/stds.htm

National Institute of Allergy and Infectious Diseases. (2004a, July). *Chlamydia*. Retrieved September 8, 2005, from http://www.niaid.nih.gov/factsheets/stdclam.htm

National Institute of Allergy and Infectious Diseases. (2004b, October). *Gonorrhea*. Retrieved September 8, 2005, from http://www.niaid.nih.gov/factsheets/stdgon.htm

Parch, L. (2003). STDs can harm babies. In L. Gerdes (Ed.), *Sexually transmitted diseases* (pp. 68–75). San Diego, CA: Greenhaven Press.

Schaffer, S.D. (2004). Vaginitis and sexually transmitted diseases. In E. Youngkin & M. Davis (Eds.), *Women's health: A primary care clinical guide* (3rd ed., pp. 261–290). Upper Saddle River, NJ: Pearson Education.

Smith, R.E., & Schaffer, S.D. (2004). Women and HIV. In E. Youngkin & M. Davis (Eds.), *Women's health: A primary care clinical guide* (3rd ed., pp. 291–302). Upper Saddle River, NJ: Pearson Education.

Resources

American Social Health Association (ASHA) (Provides education, support, and advocacy related to STI issues): www.ashastd.org

Centers for Disease Control and Prevention (CDC): www.cdc.gov

Health Check USA: www.healthcheckusa.com: Provides a list of laboratories where people can have their blood drawn for herpes tests

National Institute of Allergy and Infectious Diseases, National Institutes of Health: www.niaid.nih.gov

Planned Parenthood Federation of America: www.plannedparenthood.org

STI and AIDS hot lines

CDC: 800-342-2437 (English, 24 hours/day)
800-344-7432 (Spanish, 8 am to 2 am, 7 days/week)
800-243-7889 (TTY/Deaf access)

Herpes Resource Center: 877-411-4377
HPV and Cervical Cancer Prevention Resource Center: 877-478-5868
National Herpes Hotline (ASHA): 919-361-8488
National HPV and Cervical Cancer Prevention hot line: 919-361-4848

Chapter 11

Body Art: Tattooing, Body Piercing, and Cosmetic Tattooing

Myrna L. Armstrong, RN, EdD, FAAN

Background

Q 11.1 **Who gets tattoos and body piercings?**

Although most of the medical literature and studies tend to focus on adolescents and young adults with body art, studio artists will report that people of all ages, socioeconomic groups, genders, and occupations are obtaining tattoos and body piercings. As early as 1991 (Armstrong), artists were saying that nearly half of those obtaining tattoos were women. The latest prevalence rates for tattooing range from 19%–23%, and for body piercing the prevalence is approximately 33% (Armstrong, Roberts, Owen, & Koch, 2004). These numbers have been increasing, but there have been no national polls for a wider perspective. Overall, it seems that more men obtain tattoos, and more women obtain body piercings.

Q 11.2 **What are the health concerns with body art?**

Whether tattooing, body piercing, or cosmetic tattooing, four major concerns are present. First, no national, standardized curriculum exists to educate those performing the procedures. Anyone can open a shop and advertise for business. Kits for body piercing can be purchased for around $250 and include a procedural video plus all the equipment, complete with alcohol swabs. Tattooing for skin designs or cosmetic tattooing kits are a bit more costly because of the equipment, yet they are as easy to obtain.

Second, the invasive ingredients can be problematic. The ingredients of tattoo pigment are not standardized and are not approved by the U.S. Food and Drug Administration (FDA). Body piercing jewelry should be of high-quality surgical stainless steel, niobium, titanium, or 14-karat gold. Cosmetic jewelry can cause brass or nickel allergies. In 2004, the FDA warned of permanent makeup causing "possible disfigurements from injecting permanent ink as eyeliner, lip liner, or eyebrow coloring" (*FDA Warns of "Permanent Makeup" Scarring*, 2004).

Third, the environment in which the procedure is done can be a concern, especially when the procedure is done in homes, at flea markets, at rock concerts, at fraternity parties, or in dirty studios, where clean conditions may or may not be a priority.

Fourth, an overall lack of protection for the clientele exists. Concerns still remain about standard precautions and adequate documentation of complications. With no national regulations, states create their own, and only a few (Alaska, Oregon, and Kansas) have proposed strict, thorough legislation to protect the public undergoing the invasive procedures of tattooing, body piercing, and cosmetic tattooing. These states test the artists on anatomy, universal precautions, disease transmission, skin diseases, sterilization procedures, sanitation, personal hygiene, and aftercare instructions that are important to prevent disease or injury. These states then require mandatory continuing education. Although 36 states have changed their body-art legislation since 1998, the overall strength of the regulations still varies widely (Armstrong, 2005). For example, in some states, only a business license is required; in others, only local municipalities have regulations.

11.3   Why do people want tattoos or piercings?

Consistent studies have documented that people obtain tattoos and body piercings for self-expression and identity, something that makes them feel special and unique.

11.4   What is the average cost for a general tattoo, a body piercing, or cosmetic tattooing?

Two costs are involved with body piercings, one for the procedure and another for the jewelry (total is approximately $35–$75). Costs for a tattoo depend on the size, time needed for the design, and amount of detail associated with the figure. A 2" x 2" simplistic design costs about \$35–\$50. Cosmetic tattooing can range from \$100–\$1,200.

Q 11.5 Are people with tattoos and body piercings different than those without body art?

People typically thought to procure body art are between 15–25 years of age, and this age group tends to have higher rates of risk-taking behavior, regardless of body art. Some studies indicate that those with tattoos have even higher rates of risk-taking behavior than those with no body art (Armstrong, Owen, Roberts, & Koch, 2002a, 2002b), whereas other studies involving college students (especially with body piercing) have found that they tend to be very similar to their non–body-art counterparts (Armstrong et al., 2004).

Q 11.6 Are most people drunk when they obtain the tattooing or piercing?

Studies consistently have shown a low rate of alcohol consumption (11%–16%) before body-art procurement (Armstrong et al., 2002a, 2002b, 2004). Reputable studio artists know that alcohol increases bleeding. Marketing also is a factor. Artists know that if inebriated clients do not make good decisions, they will not be satisfied and will not return for further body art.

Q 11.7 What types of education are available for those considering getting tattoos and piercings?

Proactive discussions are important for people considering body art, but these people first should examine their own feelings (Stuppy, Armstrong, & Casals-Ariet, 1998). People who are interested in body art want applicable information. They probably already have talked with many people about tattoos and piercings and appreciate realistic material so that they have more information to make good decisions. Information from a healthcare provider can dissuade them or assist them in making good decisions as they have the actual procedure. Telling someone "no" or employing scare tactics is not realistic. Nonjudgmental communication will increase responsiveness to the information. Currently, very few audiovisual tools are available. For further information on the availability of a CD-ROM (\$25) targeted to teens and young adults, contact Texas Tech University Health Sciences Center School of Nursing, 806-743-2730.

Q 11.8   What problems can occur when people with body art have diagnostic tests such as magnetic resonance imaging (MRI)?

Recent reports from radiologic imaging, especially MRIs, have documented interaction with the heavy amount of iron-based pigments that sometimes are found in tattooing (Armstrong & Elkins, 2005). Cosmetic eye-lining can contain heavy amounts of metallic oxides of iron or titanium. As these particles are close to the skin surface, they act as conductors to deposit heat around the tattoo, creating the potential for burns and localized discomfort during the procedure. Body piercings can disperse the x-rays. People with body art should be encouraged to accurately complete any medical history surveys in the radiology department when undergoing diagnostic studies to alert staff about their tattoos and body piercings. A simple technique that healthcare providers can use to alleviate the concerns of the client's tract closing is threading sterile IV catheter tubing through the piercing site to keep the hole open during diagnostic and surgical procedures (Armstrong & Elkins).

Tattooing

Q 11.9   What is tattooing?

Using an electrically powered vertical vibrating instrument resembling a dentist's drill that uses from 1–14 solid, whisker-thin needles joined on a needle bar, tattoo pigment is injected between 50–3,000 times a minute up to or into the dermis at a depth of 1/64th to 1/16th of an inch, to create an indelible design (Armstrong & Kelly, 2001).

Q 11.10   What are the health risks related to tattooing?

Although the media portray body art as risqué and carefree behavior, both physical and psychosocial risks are associated with tattooing. Any time there are multiple punctures in the skin, the body is predisposed to infection. Hepatitis B and C are the greatest threat, as the organisms can survive on blood-contaminated surfaces for more than two months. Psychosocial risks to recipients include disappointment, low esteem, and embarrassment because they are not satisfied with the product. Some people cover their tattoos for years to avoid disclosure of their design.

Q 11.11   Can tattoos be removed?

Tattoo removal is available but is expensive, is not covered by insurance, and may take 4–12 months when trying to eliminate the design. Results depend on the pigment and location. Q-switched and pulsed lasers often are used to pulverize the pigment for removal. Small designs of black pigment are the easiest to remove. Caution is advised if a physician or technician guarantees total removal, as specific pigments and ingredients could inhibit the complete removal treatment.

Q 11.12   Is there a risk of skin cancer with tattoos?

No risk of skin cancer has been documented, but isolated cases of rare dermatologic lesions have been presented in the medical literature (Armstrong, 1991).

Q 11.13   What happens to tattoos when people get older and their skin texture changes?

As the skin ages, the design tends to broaden, turn a dull color, and lose texture and detail. After about 7–10 years, the tattoo normally fades. Some will have the design retattooed or "livened" for more color. Sunlight speeds the fading of the pigment.

Body Piercing

Q 11.14   How is a body piercing created?

Body piercing involves the insertion of sharp implements, most often large-bore hollow needles (sizes 12–16), to create an opening for decorative ornaments such as jewelry. Piercing guns should not be used for any type of piercing (including ear lobes). Studies have documented that selecting an experienced practitioner in a body-art studio is better than seeking personnel in jewelry stores or kiosks in a shopping mall (More, Seide, & Bryan, 1999). Findings include inadequate personnel training, questionable instrumentation, and poor selection of aftercare solutions. This can create difficulty in maintaining effective site care, thus predisposing the client to tract infections and embedded jewelry.

Q 11.15   What is the usual care with body piercings?

Routine care is conscientious washing of the site at least once a day with an antibacterial soap. People with body piercings need to be encouraged to start daily hygiene habits as soon as they procure the piercing. Healing times will depend on the type of piercing, location, and general care of the site. Creating a patent opening will take almost a year. Infections can happen at any time, so diligent ongoing care is a must for the duration of the piercing.

Q 11.16   If body piercings become infected, what type of care is recommended?

If an infection occurs, it initially is best to keep the jewelry in the piercing site to serve as an outlet for drainage and healing. If the jewelry is taken out, an abscess can develop in the deeper skin structures. Common culprits at the site include *Staphylococcus aureus* and *Pseudomonas aeruginosa*. If the problem does not resolve in five to seven days, the person should consult a healthcare provider for antibiotic therapy. Encourage the removal of the jewelry during the treatment period. Depending on the response to the treatment, the skin tract for the piercing jewelry could close.

Q 11.17   What are some of the most common body piercings and their health problems?

Conventional earlobe piercings are not considered body piercings because of the type of tissue and healing properties of that site. Piercings *in the ear* and *along the ear rim* are considered body piercings and are the most common type of piercings (Armstrong & Kelly, 2001). They also are the most commonly reported infected sites in the medical literature. These infections occur because auricular cartilage is less vascular, because bacteria can be introduced by the hair, or because of pressure on the ear when sleeping. Cellulitis and abscesses can develop, warranting systemic antibiotics; keloids also can form. Residual effects are scarring and site deformities, especially with high-rim cartilage piercings (Armstrong & Kelly; More et al., 1999). Navel piercings also are popular, often chosen so the person can control exposure of the piercing. This also is a site of many infections (up to 45%) because of body movement, waistband irritation, and location in a warm, moist area. Tongue piercings are popular but may modify speech or crack teeth and create a risk of aspirating the jewelry.

Q 11.18 Should body piercings be removed before surgery?

Those with body piercings are very reluctant to remove their jewelry,
especially if the piercing has just been done. Inert plastics, Teflon®
(DuPont, Wilmington, DE) posts, or retainers can be inserted to
maintain patency. These can be obtained from a local piercing shop.
If a pair of wire cutters is used to remove the shank, sharp edges are
produced on the jewelry stem, which could produce more trauma
to the piercing site when the jewelry is removed. As stated before,
threading sterile IV catheter tubing through the piercing tract can
keep the hole open for diagnostic and surgical procedures and can
alleviate the patient's concern of the tract closing (Armstrong &
Elkins, 2005).

Q 11.19 Why would anyone get an intimate body piercing (nipple and/or genitals)?

A recent study (N = 146) provides some information about this phenomenon (Caliendo, Armstrong, & Roberts, 2005). The average
age of study participants was 31, older than those with other visible
and semivisible piercings. Influences for the intimate body piercings seem to be deliberate, individual decisions stemming from an
internal motivation for sexual enhancement, self-expression, and
uniqueness. There are three different types of female genital piercings: clitoris hood, outer labia, and inner labia; males have eight
different varieties (Armstrong & Caliendo, in press).

Q 11.20 Can women with genital piercings keep their jewelry in during childbirth?

This remains a controversial topic. Although most women with
genital piercings do not believe there is any reason for concern,
healthcare providers often ask them to remove the piercing(s) for
fear of tissue tearing during the delivery. In a study by Caliendo et
al. (2005), one respondent did not remove her genital piercings
during her two pregnancies and had no ill effects (Armstrong &
Caliendo, in press).

Q 11.21 Can women with nipple piercings successfully breast-feed?

Jones (1999) asserted some interesting ideas about encouraging
those with nipple piercings to breast-feed, yet allowing retention
of their piercings. If the client has a well-healed piercing site, she

suggests a small plastic barbell so the baby can effectively clasp the nipple. Visit www.LaLecheLeague.org/FAQ/pierced.html for further information on this topic.

Cosmetic Tattooing

Q 11.22   What is cosmetic tattooing?

Permanent or cosmetic tattooing (eyeliner, eyebrows, and lip liner) is flourishing. Other names for the procedure include dermagraphics or micropigmentation. Very few articles regarding cosmetic tattooing are present in the medical literature. Application of permanent cosmetic is an invasive procedure and employs the techniques of tattooing, often using the same non–FDA-approved pigment. Cosmetic tattooing seems to need more frequent "redos" or "relivens," perhaps because of more sunlight exposure (Saunders & Armstrong, 2005).

Many states that regulate cosmetic tattooing demand adherence to the same regulations as body tattooing (Armstrong, 2005). However, women do not seem to associate permanent makeup with studio tattooing because it is marketed differently, with a focus on enhancement and radiant beauty. The results provide the same effects in the form of identity or "permanent" beauty.

Q 11.23   Where can one obtain cosmetic tattooing?

Look in the commercial pages of the telephone book under "Cosmetic Tattooing" or "Permanent Makeup." Many beauticians work out of their homes and obtain clients by word of mouth. Nationally, many cosmetologists are providing the permanent procedures, as are some nurses and physicians. Look for a reputable operator. Some operators have attended additional educational workshops to learn how to apply permanent makeup, but there is no standardization of education or instructor qualifications for the courses.

Q 11.24   Who gets cosmetic tattooing?

Women of all ages (including older adults), socioeconomic groups, and occupations are obtaining cosmetic tattooing, and the media also report some men as customers. In a recent study by Saunders and Armstrong (2005), five themes seem to unfold: (a) consistent personal "best" appearance in less time, (b) positive procedural experience, (c) admiration of other women and friends who have had the procedure done, (d) increased confidence in personal appearance, and (e) a unanimous decision to "have the procedure done again," if necessary.

Q 11.25 What are some of the risks of cosmetic tattooing?

Although complications are not commonly reported, they do arise. Complications may include imperfect application of the pigment dots, pigment migration, and procedural dissatisfaction (FDA Center for Food Safety and Applied Nutrition, 2000). Often, the beautician will have a "back-up" physician if a mistake occurs so that the error can be repaired. If the pigment is not inserted deep enough, the coloring is shed with new epidermis growth; if too deep, pigment can spread into the surrounding tissues of the eye or lips. Lip tattooing can trigger an episode of recurrent herpes. Q-switched and pulsed lasers often are used for pigment removal (Saunders & Armstrong, 2005).

References

Armstrong, M.L. (1991). Career-oriented women with tattoos. *Image: The Journal of Nursing Scholarship, 23*, 215–220.

Armstrong, M.L. (2005). Tattooing, body piercing, and permanent cosmetic state regulations: A historical and current view of state regulations with continuing concerns. *Journal of Environmental Health, 67*(8), 38–43.

Armstrong, M.L., & Caliendo, C. (in press). Genital piercings: What is known and what people with genital piercings tell us. *Urologic Nursing.*

Armstrong, M.L., & Elkins, L. (2005). Body art and MRI: Tattoos, body piercings, and permanent cosmetics may cause problems. *American Journal of Nursing, 105*(3), 65–66.

Armstrong, M.L., & Kelly, L. (2001). Tattooing, body piercing, and branding are on the rise: Perspectives for school nurses. *Journal of School Nursing, 17*, 12–23.

Armstrong, M.L., Owen, D.C., Roberts, A.E., & Koch, J.R. (2002a). College students and tattoos: The influence of image, identity, friends, and family. *Journal of Psychosocial Nursing, 40*(4), 21–29.

Armstrong, M.L., Owen, D.C., Roberts, A.E., & Koch, J.R. (2002b). College tattoos: More than skin deep. *Dermatology Nursing, 14*, 317–323.

Armstrong, M.L., Roberts, A.E., Owen, D.C., & Koch, J.R. (2004). Toward building a composite of college student influences with body art. *Issues in Comprehensive Pediatric Nursing, 27*, 273–291.

Caliendo, C., Armstrong, M.L., & Roberts, A.E. (2005). Self-reported characteristics of women and men with intimate body piercings. *Journal of Advanced Nursing, 49*, 474–484.

FDA warns of "permanent makeup" scarring. (2004, July 3). Retrieved July 4, 2004, from http://www.cnn.com/2004/HEALTH/07/02/permanent.makeup/index.html

Jones, L. (1999). Pierced nipples and breastfeeding: Achieving compromise. *Practising Midwife, 2*(11), 16–17.

More, D.R., Seide, J.L., & Bryan, P.A. (1999). Ear-piercing techniques as a cause of auricular chondritis. *Pediatric Emergency Care, 15,* 189–192.

Saunders, J.C., & Armstrong, M.L. (2005). Experiences and influences of women with cosmetic tattooing. *Dermatology Nursing, 17,* 23–31.

Stuppy, D.J., Armstrong, M.L., & Casals-Ariet, C. (1998). Attitudes of health care providers and students towards tattooed people. *Journal of Advanced Nursing, 27,* 1165–1170.

U.S. Food and Drug Administration Center for Food Safety and Applied Nutrition. (2000, November 29). *Tattoos and permanent makeup* [Office of Cosmetics and Colors fact sheet]. Retrieved January 13, 2003, from http://vm.cfsan.fda.gov/~dms/cos-204.html

Resource

Texas Tech University Health Sciences Center School of Nursing offers a CD-ROM on "Body Art Education" ($25) 806-743-2730.

Chapter 12

Smoking and Smoking Cessation

Lori Kondas, BA, RRT, CPFT, AE-C

Background

Q 12.1 Why should I stop smoking?

Tobacco use is the number-one preventable cause of death in the United States. Cigarette smoking kills 178,000 women in the United States annually (American Lung Association [ALA], 2004). The major causes of death are lung cancer (44,000), heart disease (41,000), and chronic lung disease (37,500). Lung cancer deaths alone have risen approximately 600% in the past 60 years (Centers for Disease Control and Prevention [CDC], 2004b). Smoking harms nearly every part of the body, causing many diseases and reducing the health of smokers in general. CDC (2004a) has listed these effects on particular parts of the body.

Cardiovascular system: Women who smoke greatly increase their risk of heart disease, including stroke, heart attack, vascular disease, and aneurysm. Smoking causes blood vessels to become narrow and blocked. A combination of increased cholesterol levels and blood clots inside the blood vessels increases the risk of heart attack and death. Cigarette smoking has been associated with sudden cardiac death of all types in both men and women. When the blood vessels in the brain are affected, an increased risk of stroke occurs.

Respiratory system: All of the toxic gases inhaled when a person smokes damage the lungs. In addition to lung cancer, smoking causes other lung diseases such as chronic bronchitis and emphysema. Smoking is directly responsible for 80% of chronic obstructive pulmonary disease (COPD) deaths in women. More women than men die from COPD every year (ALA, 2004). For people with asthma, smoking triggers asthma symptoms, and it increases both the number and severity of asthma episodes.

Digestive system: Smoking has harmful effects on all parts of the digestive system, contributing to such common problems as heartburn and peptic ulcers. Smoking can cause more frequent and severe episodes of heartburn. Smokers have a higher risk of ulcers, and the ulcers of smokers tend to heal slower than ulcers in non-smokers. Smoking increases the risk of Crohn disease and possibly gallstones. Smoking seems to affect the liver, too, by changing the way it handles drugs and alcohol.

Musculoskeletal system: Smoking is a risk factor for osteoporosis and bone fractures. Fractures take longer to heal in smokers because of the harmful effects of nicotine on the production of bone-forming cells. Smoking also is associated with lower-back pain and rheumatoid arthritis.

Reproductive health: Cigarette smoking has harmful effects on the ability both to become pregnant and to carry a pregnancy to term. Pregnant smokers are more likely to have low-birthweight babies and premature birth. The rates of sudden infant death syndrome are higher in a household where someone smokes.

Other effects: According to the National Institute on Drug Abuse (NIDA, 2005), smokers are more than twice as likely as nonsmokers to develop Alzheimer disease. They also have two to three times the risk of developing cataracts, the leading cause of blindness and visual loss, as nonsmokers. Smoking lessens one's normal life expectancy by an average of 13–15 years. Smoking causes wrinkles by reducing blood flow to the skin and decreases the amount of vitamins in the skin.

Smoking also can affect the health of nonsmokers. The same cancer-causing chemicals found in inhaled tobacco smoke are found in secondhand tobacco smoke. Nonsmokers exposed to secondhand smoke are at increased risk for lung cancer and coronary heart disease, and children exposed to tobacco smoke have elevated risks of ear infections and respiratory infections (NIDA, 2001).

Q 12.2   How long does it take cigarette smoking to harm a smoker?

Many people believe they can smoke for a long time before smoking will hurt them. The truth is that the first puff of the first cigarette causes damage to the body. Every single puff of a cigarette increases heart and breathing rates, constricts blood vessels, and decreases the oxygen-carrying capacity in the blood. Smoking also is highly addictive. The first symptoms of nicotine dependence can appear within days to weeks of the beginning of occasional use, often even before daily smoking occurs.

Not only does cigarette smoke instantly cause harm to the smoker, but it also has immediate effects on everyone within breathing distance. Environmental tobacco smoke is classified as a group A carcinogen, a category used when there is clear evidence of cancer-causing agents in humans (U.S. Department of Health and Human Services, 2005).

Q 12.3   How can cigarettes cause so many different problems?

When smoke is inhaled, it is carried deep into the lungs, where it is absorbed quickly into the bloodstream and carried throughout the entire body. One chemical found in tobacco smoke is nicotine. Nicotine affects many systems in the body, including the heart and blood vessels, the hormonal system, the body's metabolism, and the brain.

Q 12.4   Once I stop smoking, can I still smoke a cigarette now and then?

There is no safe amount of tobacco. Even one cigarette can cause harm to the body. To add to the problem, when an ex-smoker smokes a cigarette, even years after quitting, the addictive properties of nicotine may be triggered, quickly causing the person to want to smoke more. Many people relapse with the thought that they can smoke just one cigarette. Just as an alcoholic should not take another drink, a former smoker should avoid cigarettes at all times.

Q 12.5   What kinds of cancer are caused by smoking?

Cigarette smoking is the major cause of lung cancer among women. In 1987, lung cancer surpassed breast cancer to become the leading cause of cancer deaths among women (CDC, 2004b).

Unfortunately, lung cancer is not the only cancer linked to smoking. Smoking also is associated with cancers of the mouth, pharynx, larynx, esophagus, stomach, pancreas, cervix, kidney, and bladder, as well as some forms of leukemia. The overall rates of death from cancer are twice as high among smokers as among nonsmokers, with heavy smokers having rates that are four times greater than those of nonsmokers. Cigarette smoking is the most important preventable cause of cancer in the United States.

12.6 What harmful chemicals are found in cigarettes?

More than 4,000 different chemical compounds have been identified in tobacco smoke (U.S. Department of Health and Human Services, 2005). Of these, at least 60 are known to cause cancer, and hundreds are considered toxic chemicals. Some of these chemicals occur naturally in the tobacco leaf, and some are created when tobacco is burned. Manufacturers also add chemicals to make cigarettes milder and easier to inhale, to improve taste, and to prolong burning and shelf life. Some of the chemicals found in tobacco are also in wood varnish, the insect poison DDT, arsenic, nail polish remover, and rat poison. The following are examples of some of the chemicals found in cigarette smoke.
- Ammonia (a chemical used to clean toilets)
- Arsenic (a poison used to kill insects or weeds)
- Benzene (a flammable, toxic liquid used as a solvent or motor fuel)
- Cyanide (a poison used to kill rats)
- Formaldehyde (a chemical used to preserve dead frogs)
- Hydrazine (a corrosive liquid used in fuels for rockets and jets)
- Nicotine (a pesticide used to kill insects)
- Phenol (a poisonous compound used as a disinfectant)
- Styrene (a liquid used in making synthetic rubber and plastics)
- Toluene (a liquid used as an antiknock agent in gasoline)

12.7 Is cigarette smoking a bad habit or an addiction?

Tobacco contains nicotine, a chemical that causes physical addiction to smoking and makes it difficult for people to stop smoking. In fact, nicotine is recognized as one of the most frequently used addictive drugs. From the first cigarette, inhaling nicotine results in an almost immediate "kick," but this high does not last. If the person does not smoke for a few hours, the level of nicotine in the body begins to fall. As the level of nicotine drops, the smoker experiences cravings and other symptoms of withdrawal. In an effort to temporarily stop the symptoms of withdrawal, the smoker needs to increase the level of nicotine in the body. This is when the smoker lights up the next cigarette. Eventually, the brain becomes dependent on nicotine, and the smoker becomes an addicted user.

Once the addiction sets in, smokers begin to create new associations or habits around smoking. Over time, patterns are formed as smokers begin to associate everyday actions with smoking. These might include having a cup of coffee, being tense or worried, talking on the phone, driving, taking a break at work, having a drink, being with friends, or just wanting something to do with their hands. People should address both the addiction and the everyday actions associated with smoking in order to successfully stop smoking.

12.8   Why is it so hard to stop smoking?

Once people become physically addicted to the nicotine that is found in all tobacco products, they only feel comfortable when it is in their bodies. After several tobacco-free hours, the uncomfortable symptoms of withdrawal set in.

Quitting also is hard because cigarettes are a big part of a smoker's life. Smokers may enjoy holding cigarettes and inhaling the smoke. They may light a cigarette when they feel stressed, bored, or angry. In addition, after months and years of lighting up, smoking becomes part of their daily routine. Smokers may light up automatically without even thinking about it. They feel pleasure or reduced tension when they smoke. This constant reinforcement makes it harder for a person to stop smoking for good.

12.9   Is any type of tobacco safe?

No safe tobacco product exists; all types of tobacco are dangerous. The use of any tobacco product—including cigarettes, cigars, pipes, spit tobacco, mentholated, "low tar," "naturally grown," or "additive free"—can cause cancer and other adverse health effects.

Pipe and cigar smokers significantly increase their risk of disease and death. Pipe smokers have a very high rate of lip cancer, and compared to cigarette smokers, pipe and cigar smokers have a higher chance of getting mouth cancer, throat cancer, and larynx (voice box) cancer.

Some people think that smokeless tobacco is safer than cigarettes, but this is not true. This form of tobacco is as addictive as cigarettes and can cause many damaging health effects, including an increased risk of cancer of the mouth and pharynx.

Some people think that switching from high-tar and high-nicotine cigarettes to those with lower levels of tar and nicotine makes smoking safer, but this is not true. When people switch to brands with lower tar and nicotine, they often end up smoking more cigarettes, or more of each cigarette, to get the same nicotine dose as before. Smoking cigarettes with lower machine-measured yields of tar and nicotine provides no clear benefit to health.

Cessation Interventions

Q 12.10   What medications or products can I use to help me to quit smoking?

Using medication can greatly increase a smoker's chance of successfully quitting. Nicotine replacement treatment, combined with psychological support and skills training to avoid relapse, results in some of the highest long-term smoking cessation rates (U.S. Public Health Service, 2000).

Nicotine replacement products help to relieve some of the withdrawal symptoms people experience when they quit smoking. Several types of nicotine replacement products are available that are safe and effective; these include the nicotine patch, nicotine nasal spray, nicotine gum, nicotine inhaler, and nicotine lozenges. Proper use of replacement products and prescription medications is described in the *Quick Reference Guide for Clinicians* (Fiore et al., 2000) from the U.S. Department of Health and Human Services.

One medication that can help people to stop smoking is bupropion (Zyban®, GlaxoSmithKline, Research Triangle Park, NC). This is not a nicotine replacement, as are the gum and patch. Instead, this medication works by helping the former smoker control nicotine craving or thoughts about cigarette use. The drug, available by prescription only, also is sold as an antidepressant under the name Wellbutrin® (GlaxoSmithKline).

Common side effects are dry mouth, difficulty sleeping, dizziness, and skin rash. People should not use this drug if they have a seizure condition such as epilepsy or an eating disorder such as anorexia nervosa or bulimia, or if they are taking other medicines that contain bupropion hydrochloride.

Q 12.11   What is nicotine replacement therapy?

Nicotine replacement therapies are used to relieve withdrawal symptoms. Products such as the nicotine patch, nasal spray, gum, inhaler, and lozenges can help women work on the "habit" and "social" parts of quitting first, while gradually reducing the amount of nicotine used over time. An added benefit is that these products do not contain the cancer-causing chemicals associated with tobacco smoke.

Pregnant women or those with heart problems should be sure to talk to their healthcare provider before using nicotine replacement therapy. Some nicotine replacement products require a prescription; gum and patches can be bought without one. With all types of nicotine replacement therapy, it is necessary to follow the healthcare provider's guidance and use these products only as prescribed and/or according to labeling.

Nicotine replacement products deliver small, steady doses of nicotine into the body, which helps to relieve the withdrawal symptoms often felt by people trying to quit smoking. Refer to Fiore et al. (2000) or Agency for Healthcare Research and Quality (2005) for specific product information and use.

The **nicotine patch** supplies a steady amount of nicotine to the body through the skin. The nicotine patch is sold in varying strengths. It may not be a good choice for people with skin problems or allergies to adhesive tape.

Nicotine gum is available in strengths of 2 and 4 mg. Chewing nicotine gum releases nicotine into the bloodstream through the lining of the mouth. Nicotine gum might not be appropriate for people with temporomandibular joint disease or for those with dentures or other dental work.

Nicotine nasal spray comes in a pump bottle containing nicotine that tobacco users can inhale when they have an urge to smoke. This product is not recommended for people with nasal or sinus conditions, allergies, or asthma.

Nicotine inhaler devices deliver a vaporized form of nicotine to the mouth through a mouthpiece attached to a plastic cartridge. Anyone with a severe reactive airway disease should check with his or her doctor before using this product.

Nicotine lozenges come in the form of a hard "candy" and release nicotine as they slowly dissolve in the mouth. They are available in strengths of 2 and 4 mg. Lozenges should not be chewed or swallowed.

Q 12.12   I am concerned about gaining weight when I quit. What can I do to avoid weight gain?

The average weight gain after quitting smoking usually is less than 10 pounds and can be controlled through diet and exercise. To avoid weight gain, new nonsmokers should eat a healthy diet and stay active. Before quitting, women should have plenty of low-calorie snacks in the house so they are not tempted to fill up on high-calorie junk food when cravings hit. For some people, eating smaller, more frequent meals also will prevent weight gain. Avoiding boredom and finding ways to keep busy also may eliminate the tendency to gain weight after quitting.

Increasing activity will reduce the chance of weight gain and will increase the chance of long-term success. Women who are not physically active have a greater risk of gaining weight after quitting than active women. An exercise program can reduce or delay weight gain after cessation and can increase the quit rate among women. Women should try to get 30 minutes or more of moderate-intensity physical activity on most days of the week, preferably every day.

Q 12.13   What are the most effective methods for women to stop smoking?

As noted earlier, pharmacologic treatment combined with behavior modification, including support and skills training, results in some of the highest long-term abstinence rates. Women who have a strong commitment to change, take the time to learn new coping skills, and use social support are more likely to succeed in quitting. Smokers should find out what resources are available and take advantage of smoking cessation classes or supportive programs. Getting family, friends, and coworkers to support the quit attempt will increase the chance of success. Following five basic steps will help smokers quit for good.

- Start by setting a quit date and getting rid of all cigarettes, lighters, and ashtrays.
- Get support and encouragement from family and friends, and consider signing up for a class or support group.
- Learn new skills and behaviors. People trying to quit should think about the situations that make them want a cigarette and plan other options for when those situations arise.

- Get medication, and use it correctly.
- Be prepared for relapse or difficult situations.

Q 12.14   I have tried to quit before and it did not work. What can I do?

Quitting smoking is hard. For some women, it takes a few tries before they are finally able to quit for good. The most important thing is to learn from the unsuccessful attempt. Identifying the reasons one went back to smoking can be the basis of an effective smoking cessation plan. Once potential relapse situations are identified, the person can look for new ways to handle these situations in ways that do not involve smoking.

Before lighting the final cigarette, it is important to spend some time planning. First, people should learn what things trigger or cause them to smoke. Next, smokers should plan options for dealing with these triggers. Using nicotine replacement therapy also may increase the chance for success. Generally, rates of relapse for smoking cessation are highest in the first few weeks and months and diminish considerably after about three months.

Q 12.15   What is smoking withdrawal like?

The symptoms of withdrawal are actually signs that the body is recovering from the effects of smoking. Although these may be unpleasant, they do get better, and eventually they should go away. Common withdrawal signs include nausea, headache, constipation, diarrhea, increased appetite, drowsiness, fatigue, insomnia, inability to concentrate, irritability, hostility, anxiety, depression, and craving for tobacco. Not every person experiences all of these, but it is helpful to know how the body might react to life without cigarettes.

Using nicotine replacement therapy or bupropion may help to avoid some of these withdrawal symptoms. Learning new ways to deal with stress, joining a smoking cessation program or support group, and adding an exercise program also can help new nonsmokers cope with withdrawal.

Q 12.16   What happens to my body when I quit?

Quitting smoking has immediate as well as long-term benefits, reducing risks for diseases caused by smoking and improving health in general. The benefits of quitting smoking are great. Within 20 minutes of smoking the last cigarette, the body begins to restore itself. For example, after only 24 hours, the chance of a heart attack decreases. The excess risk of developing heart disease as a result of smoking may be reduced by as much as half in the year or two after quitting. After 15 years, the former smoker's risk of heart disease and stroke approaches that of a person who has never smoked (American Heart Association, 2005). Women who quit smoking by age 35 increase their life expectancy by six to eight years.

Quitting smoking reduces the risk of lung cancer. Ten years after quitting, the risk for lung cancer is 30%–50% that of the risk of those who continue to smoke. Although the risk of developing lung cancer declines after smoking cessation, the risk remains higher than that of never-smokers (CDC, 2004b).

It is never too late to gain benefits from quitting! Quitting at age 45 increases life expectancy by six or seven years. Quitting at age 55 increases life expectancy by three to six years. Quitting at age 65 increases life expectancy by 1.4–4 years (CDC, 2004b).

Health Considerations

12.17   Some of my friends and family are smokers. Even though I do not smoke, can secondhand smoke harm my health?

Although people often think of the medical consequences that result from direct use of tobacco products, passive or secondary smoke also increases the risk for many diseases. Significant numbers of people die from secondhand smoke each year in the United States, as well. Exposure to secondhand smoke is a cause of lung cancer among women who have never smoked. Contact with a spouse's secondhand smoke is a cause of death from heart disease among women who do not smoke.

Exposure to tobacco smoke in the home increases the severity of asthma, and it is a risk factor for new cases of childhood asthma. Additionally, dropped cigarettes are the leading cause of house fire fatalities, leading to more than 1,000 deaths each year.

12.18   Is it safe to smoke when taking birth control pills or when using a birth control patch?

No. If women smoke cigarettes and also take oral contraceptives, they are more prone to heart attacks and stroke than other smokers; this especially is true for women older than 35. Women who use oral contraceptives should be strongly advised not to smoke.

12.19   Can smoking affect my ability to get pregnant?

Women who smoke are at an increased risk for infertility, complications during pregnancy, and an earlier onset of menopause.

12.20   What happens if I smoke during my pregnancy?

The chemicals in tobacco smoke will be passed on to a mother's unborn baby and can harm her baby even before she knows she is pregnant. Women who smoke during pregnancy increase the risk of pregnancy complications, premature delivery, low-birthweight infants, stillbirth, and sudden infant death syndrome. The harmful effects of smoking may occur in every trimester of pregnancy; they range from spontaneous abortions in the first trimester to increased premature delivery rates and decreased birth weights in the final trimester. Mothers' smoking during pregnancy reduces their babies' lung function after birth.

In pregnant women, smoking interferes with the oxygen supply to the baby. Nicotine easily crosses the placenta, and nicotine concentrations in the fetus can be higher than in the mother. It appears that nicotine is concentrated in fetal blood, amniotic fluid, and breast milk. Another ingredient of tobacco smoke, carbon monoxide, has been shown to inhibit the release of oxygen into fetal tissues (Youngkin & Davis, 2004).

12.21   Why do most people start to smoke?

Nearly all first uses of tobacco occur before age 18, and because nicotine is addictive, adolescents who smoke regularly are likely to become adult smokers. The influence of friends and peers and curiosity are the major reasons young people try smoking. In addition, people with friends and parents who smoke are more likely to begin smoking than those who have nonsmoking parents. Those who begin to smoke at a younger age are more likely than late starters to develop long-term nicotine addiction.

Advertising and promotion of tobacco products also affect the likelihood that someone will start smoking. The tobacco industry spends billions of dollars each year to create and distribute ads that show smoking as an exciting, glamorous, healthy adult activity.

12.22   Is it harder for women to stop smoking?

Large-scale smoking cessation trials show that women are less likely to try to quit and may be more likely to relapse if they quit (NIDA, 2001). In cessation programs using nicotine replacement methods, such as the patch or gum, the nicotine does not seem to reduce cravings as effectively for women as for men. Other factors that may contribute to women's difficulty with quitting are the facts that the withdrawal symptoms may be more intense for women and that they appear more likely than men to gain weight upon quitting. Learning new methods for dealing with stress, finding strong social support, and starting an exercise program can help women overcome these obstacles.

12.23   What is the best way to help someone to quit smoking?

The decision to quit smoking must start with the smoker; never try to push anyone into stopping. The best way to provide support is to be a good listener. Let the smoker talk, and do not be tempted to preach or offer too much advice. Give him or her the chance to talk about problems, and provide support through any crisis that may increase the urge to start smoking again. If the person has a slip, help him or her to recognize what went wrong, and then assist in planning to help the person avoid relapse in the future. Plan activities to help the person stay busy, and offer smoke-free company. Above all, be supportive. Sometimes just "being there" is the best way to help.

12.24   How can healthcare providers help their patients to stop smoking?

Healthcare providers can be good sources of information about the health risks of smoking and about quitting. They can tell their patients about the proper use and potential side effects of nicotine replacement therapy and help them to find local smoking cessation programs.

Healthcare providers also can play an important role by *asking* patients about smoking at every office visit; *advising* patients to stop; *assessing* readiness and willingness to quit; *assisting* patients by setting a quit date, providing self-help materials, and suggesting nicotine replacement therapies (when appropriate); and *arranging* for follow-up visits. The Ask, Advise, Assess, Assist, and Arrange model was developed to help healthcare professionals manage their patients who smoke (Agency for Healthcare Research and Quality, 2005). People who have even a brief counseling session with a healthcare professional are more likely to quit smoking.

Q 12.25   What agencies and organizations are available to help people to stop smoking?

Many different organizations offer information, counseling, and other services on how to quit as well as information on where to go for help. Make sure to go to a reliable, credible source for assistance. The agencies listed in Table 12-1 are good places to start.

Table 12-1. Cessation Resources

Organization/Program	Phone Number	Web Site
American Cancer Society	800-ACS-2345	www.cancer.org
American Heart Association	800-AHA-USA-1 (800-242-8721)	www.americanheart.org
American Lung Association	800-LUNG-USA (800-586-4872)	www.lungusa.org
Centers for Disease Control and Prevention Office on Smoking and Health	800-CDC-1311 (800-232-1311)	www.cdc.gov/tobacco
National Cancer Institute Cancer Information Service	800-4-CANCER (800-422-6237)	www.cancer.gov/tobacco
National Women's Health Information Center	800-994-9662 888-220-5446 for the hearing impaired	www.4woman.gov

References

Agency for Healthcare Research and Quality. (2005, March). *Helping smokers quit: A guide for nurses.* Rockville, MD: Author. Retrieved September 6, 2005, from http://www.ahrq.gov/about/nursing/hlpsmksqt.htm

American Heart Association. (2005). *Smoking cessation.* Retrieved September 6, 2005, from http://www.americanheart.org/presenter.jhtml?identifier=4731

American Lung Association. (2004, November). *Women and smoking fact sheet.* Retrieved September 6, 2005, from http://www.lungusa.org/site/pp.asp?c=dvLUK9O0E&b=33572

Centers for Disease Control and Prevention. (2004a). *The health consequences of smoking: A report of the surgeon general.* Retrieved September 6, 2005, from http://www.cdc.gov/tobacco/sgr/sgr_2004/

Centers for Disease Control and Prevention. (2004b, May). *Women and tobacco fact sheet.* Retrieved September 6, 2005, from http://www.cdc.gov/tobacco/factsheets/WomenTobacco_Factsheet.htm

Fiore, M.C., Bailey, W.C., Cohen, S.J., Dorfman, S.F., Goldstein, M.G., Gritz, E.R., et al. (2000, October). *Treating tobacco use and dependence. Quick reference guide for clinicians.* Rockville, MD: U.S. Department of Health and Human Services. Retrieved September 6, 2005, from http://www.surgeongeneral.gov/tobacco/tobaqrg.htm

National Institute on Drug Abuse. (2001). *Nicotine addiction* (NIH Publication No. 01-4342). Retrieved September 6, 2005, from http://www.drugabuse.gov/researchreports/nicotine/nicotine.html

National Institute on Drug Abuse. (2005). *NIDA InfoFacts: Cigarettes and other nicotine products.* Retrieved September 6, 2005, from http://www.drugabuse.gov/infofacts/tobacco.html

U.S. Department of Health and Human Services. (2005, April). *Report on Carcinogens* (11th ed.). Retrieved March 13, 2006, from http://ntp.niehs.nih.gov/ntp/roc/toc11.html

U.S. Public Health Service. (2000, June). *Treating tobacco use and dependence: Summary.* Retrieved September 6, 2005, from http://www.surgeongeneral.gov/tobacco/smokesum.htm

Youngkin, E., & Davis, M. (2004). Assessing women's health. In E. Youngkin & M. Davis (Eds.), *Women's health: A primary care clinical guide* (3rd ed., pp. 53–102). Upper Saddle River, NJ: Pearson Education.

Resources

Agency for Health Care Research and Quality: www.ahrq.gov/consumer/index.html#smoking

Cessation Resource Center: http://apps.nccd.cdc.gov/crc

National Cancer Institute quit line: 877-44U-QUIT; smoking cessation Web site: www.smokefree.gov

Nicotine Anonymous: www.nicotine-anonymous.org

Professional Assisted Cessation Therapy™: www.endsmoking.org

Smokefree.gov: www.smokefree.gov

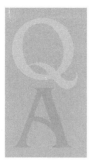

Chapter 13
Eating Disorders

Ellen Homlong, RD, LD, CDE

Background

13.1 What is an eating disorder?

An eating disorder is the result of a drive for thinness and a morbid dread of body fat. This results in an obsession with weight and a preoccupation with foods, coupled with marked irrational thoughts and a clear disturbance in how people view themselves and their bodies. Diet restrictions and eating patterns are self-imposed, and people with eating disorders typically are in denial of the seriousness of their eating habits.

13.2 What is the prevalence of eating disorders?

Conservative estimates in the United States indicate that after puberty, 10 million girls and women and 1 million boys and men are struggling with an eating disorder such as anorexia or bulimia, and up to an additional 25 million are dealing with binge-eating conditions (National Eating Disorders Association [NEDA], 2002b). Because of the secretiveness and shame associated with disordered eating, many cases probably are not reported. Also, many normal dieters will progress to disordered eating, joining the many millions of girls and women who are dissatisfied with their bodies.

13.3 What is the difference between anorexia and bulimia?

Anorexia nervosa is the self-imposed restriction of foods, thus denying the body essential nutrients. Bulimia manifests itself in apparently normal eating patterns followed by purging. Many bulimics also secretly consume large food quantities with subsequent purging. Both conditions share common distorted beliefs, feelings of shame, being "out of control," and guilt after food intake and/or purging. In both anorexia and bulimia, common "hunger" and "fullness" cues are not recognized. At some point, a person with an eating disorder may display signs of both anorexia and bulimia. Both conditions may exist together or separately throughout the duration of the eating disorder.

 13.4   Is binge eating also an eating disorder?

Binge eating is a newly recognized eating disorder. The eating pattern is characterized by frequent episodes of uncontrolled and excessive food intake over a short time period. Binge-eating disorder shares many characteristics with bulimia, such as the secrecy of food intake, feelings of guilt and disgust after a binge, and the lack of regard to hunger and fullness cues. A binge eater does not purge after food intake and is more likely to develop some of the health risks associated with obesity, such as diabetes, heart disease, and high blood pressure.

 13.5   Do people who eat nonfood items have an eating disorder?

Many problem conditions exist that involve food, eating, and weight. The condition referred to in this situation is called "pica," a craving for nonfood items such as dirt, chalk, paint chips, and rubber. Other conditions displaying disordered eating behavior include night-eating syndrome, Prader-Willi syndrome (a metabolic pituitary condition), chewing and spitting, and compulsive exercising (anorexia athletica). These are less-well-known eating disorders and often lack official diagnosis.

Symptoms

 13.6   How will I know if someone has an eating disorder?

Clearly, it can be challenging to recognize an eating disorder, as dieting and weight concerns have become a norm. How would one know when the behavior is so abnormal it threatens a person's emotional and physical health? Warning signs include consistent refusal of foods, fast and significant weight loss (anorexia), excuses not to eat ("just ate," "not hungry"), and avoidance of favorite foods. Commonly, the person shows a significant interest in food and cooking, without eating any of the foods prepared or only taking tiny portions. Nutrition labels are religiously studied, and only low- or no-fat foods are consumed. A characteristic of bulimia is the person's disappearance to the bathroom or other hiding place immediately after a meal. Weight loss may not be significant or noticeable in a person with bulimia.

13.7   My mother, who is 85 years old, has lost a lot of weight. Her physician just diagnosed her with anorexia. Does she really have an eating disorder?

The mother in this case does not have an eating disorder, as in anorexia nervosa, which is a psychiatric condition. Her anorexia implies that she is malnourished because of appetite loss and possibly lack of smell and taste. These are unfortunate but common characteristics of the aging process. The daughter should talk to her mother's physician or a dietitian about her mother's diet and medical conditions. They will assist her mother with strategies to improve her nutrition intake.

13.8   My friend has lost a lot of weight, and she is not very interested in social activities anymore. Should I be concerned?

Yes, this situation presents reasons to be concerned. The person has observed two very common signs of an eating disorder. The earlier this is addressed, the better the chances are for a quick recovery. If a woman suspects her friend has an eating disorder, she should assure her friend that she can be trusted and ask her questions about her life to open up a dialogue. The friend may be resistant at first to talk about her weight and relationship with food. If the person is unable to make any progress, she should talk to someone she feels she can trust with her suspicion. It is important that her friend feels safe with her. However, a person never should promise her friend that she will keep her eating disorder a secret. Professionals who can treat eating disorders have to become involved, and the person in this case may be a vital link to ensure that this step is taken. The friend may admit to the problem yet try to maintain secrecy and resist treatment.

Recovery/Treatment

13.9   I know someone who has struggled with an eating disorder for more than 10 years. What are the chances of recovery?

The longer a person has struggled with an eating disorder, the longer and more difficult the recovery process.

13.10   What type of treatment is available for someone with an eating disorder?

The treatment options for someone with an eating disorder depend on the type as well as the severity and duration of the illness. Equally important is the person's readiness to face recovery. Many eating disorder clients recover successfully in an outpatient setting with supervision and counseling from a medical doctor, mental health professional, and dietitian. Others are not so fortunate and will have to commit to a more rigid recovery program in an inpatient setting. Both treatment options may take weeks, months, or even years to complete. However, the end result is what matters—a healthy body image and new eating habits that recognize hunger and fullness cues as well as favorite foods, regardless of calorie content.

13.11   How do I know what type of treatment is necessary for an individual with an eating disorder?

An assessment by a healthcare professional specializing in eating disorders will determine the best and most effective treatment options for each specific case. This professional also will assist in the choice of facility as needed. Geographic location, cost, and convenience are major considerations when selecting an eating disorder treatment program. Unfortunately, some health insurance policies do not recognize the need for options. The individual's insurance coverage may be the deciding factor in dictating treatment options.

13.12   How do I ensure that an individual with an eating disorder will be getting the best care possible?

Because the recovery process in most cases is very slow, a person cannot expect to see immediate results. How an individual responds to treatment will vary greatly. However, if a person suspects minimal progress is being made after months of therapy, he or she should talk to the professional working with the person being treated. The individual suffering from an eating disorder may not be truthful in reporting progress, as denial and resistance to recovery are common. If the individual is older than 18 years of age, others will need her permission in order to discuss the progress with her therapist(s).

Sadly, many victims of eating disorders do not seek appropriate care from healthcare professionals with expertise in the area of eating disorders. They may rely on a family doctor and/or generalized psychologist to treat the illness. This person may not be equipped to take on someone with an eating disorder. Suggesting a second opinion may be an option if someone is concerned that the person he or she cares about is not getting better.

13.13 I suspect my daughter has an eating disorder, and she has been grounded until she eats more and gains back the weight she lost. Is there anything else I can do?

The concerns of a mother in such a situation are understandable, and her feelings of helplessness certainly are validated. If a mother suspects her daughter of having an eating disorder, has the mother provided an opportunity for them to talk about her observations and ruled out any medical causes for the weight loss? If the daughter has an eating disorder, she probably will find a way to continue practicing her behavior, and punishment measures may cause more harm than good by building defiance. It would be helpful to take the daughter to see a physician specializing in adolescent medicine as soon as possible. The mother should provide her daughter with unconditional support and listen to her without judgment.

13.14 Are some women at greater risk for developing eating disorders?

Because of the continuous demand for thinness, certain populations are at a greater risk for developing an eating disorder. This includes models, cheerleaders, dancers, runners, and other athletes. Females who develop anorexia often were "good children," eager to please and avoid conflict. They want to be special and strive for perfection. People who become bulimic often have problems with control of impulses, anxiety, and depression. Many women who develop eating disorders have experienced physical, emotional, or sexual abuse. Low self-esteem is almost certain among populations with anorexia, bulimia, and binge-eating disorder (NEDA, 2002a).

13.15 Are adolescent females the only group at risk for developing eating disorders?

The prevalence of eating disorders favors adolescent females; however, a growing number of males now are being recognized as a population at risk. The onset of an eating disorder seems to strike young girls at an increasingly earlier age. Girls express the desire to be thinner as early as first grade, and 81% of 10-year-olds are afraid of being fat (NEDA, 2002b). A binge-eating disorder is more prevalent among females at various ages, and many "normal dieters" progress to pathologic dieting. This can occur at any age.

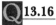 **13.16** **What are some of the medical consequences for a person with anorexia?**

Anorexia nervosa should be viewed as a life-threatening disorder. Depending on the severity and duration of the disorder, 5%–20% of those with anorexia nervosa will die (American Psychiatric Association, 2000). Health consequences include severe dehydration, fatigue, and depletion of muscle mass. Often, an abnormally slow heart rate develops as heart muscle also is lost. Hair and skin are generally dry. A layer of downy, fine hair may grow on different parts of the body in an effort to keep the body warm, now that fat stores are depleted and no longer serve as insulation. Amenorrhea (loss of three consecutive menstrual periods) is common, and some women may suffer irreversible infertility problems (Martin, 2004).

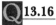 **13.17** **My friend has admitted she is bulimic. She has not lost any weight, and I never see her gorging on foods. Could she be making this up?**

Kudos to the friend for admitting she has a difficult relationship with food. Because most people with bulimia maintain weight and may even gain some weight in spite of purging habits, others will not see the drastic physical changes common with anorexia. The bingeing and purging pattern of a bulimic typically is kept secret. Chances are the friend will eat normally when she is with other people and look for opportunities to gorge in private. A person may notice that her friend will visit the bathroom almost immediately after a meal or make excuses to leave others' company after a meal. This will be a good time to talk to her about her thoughts and feelings and assist her in a recovery program. The friend in this situation has taken the first step toward recovery by admitting she has a problem.

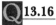 **13.18** **If there are no physical signs of bulimia, could my friend still have medical problems as a result?**

Eating disorders can affect every cell in a person's body. Although bulimia may not display the obvious physical changes common in anorexia, this condition is not exempt from physical manifestations. Common medical problems are destruction of teeth, rupture of the esophagus, and swollen neck glands because of persistent vomiting. Laxative users also may suffer dependency and permanent intestinal damage because of abuse of these remedies. In addition, those with bulimia and anorexia share the risks of osteoporosis, infertility, organ damage, and a weakened immune system.

Q 13.19   My teenage daughter has just started treatment for anorexia, and the dietitian is asking her to eat 1,200 calories per day. Can this possibly be enough calories?

It is a start. Most people with anorexia eat far less. Although the daughter in this case will need much more than this to sustain good health, asking her to eat more than 1,200 calories initially may be self-defeating. If the patient can feel comfortable eating 1,200 calories per day, the dietitian will work with her to expel myths and fears about foods and calories. The more comfortable this person becomes with food and her body image, the easier it will be to introduce new foods and a greater amount of calories. Be patient. She is on the right track to recovery.

Q 13.20   My daughter is seeing a dietitian to help her to overcome food fears, as she has been diagnosed with anorexia. Her physician is insisting she also should see a therapist for psychological counseling. Is this really necessary?

Absolutely. Anorexia, as well as other eating disorders, is a psychological disorder. Recovery will not be possible without addressing the underlying issues related to the abnormal eating patterns and distorted body image. Ask the dietitian or physician about a referral to a therapist with experience and academic background related to eating disorders. Make sure the therapist, physician, and dietitian have ongoing communication and an open dialogue regarding the patient's progress.

Q 13.21   Are eating disorders classified as a medical or psychiatric condition?

Eating disorders arise from a combination of longstanding social and psychological conditions. Troubled interpersonal relationships often tied to family dynamics may contribute to feelings of loneliness, inadequacy, and depression. Out of this grows the desire to be "special" and an intense need for control. Dieting, bingeing, and purging undermine health but help some people to numb painful emotions and provide them with a sense of control over their lives. The consequences of this behavior ultimately cause medical problems; however, it is a person's psychological disposition that triggers the onset of an eating disorder.

References

American Psychiatric Association. (2000). *Diagnostic and statistical manual of mental disorders* (4th ed., text rev.). Washington, DC: Author.

Martin, A. (2004). Psychosocial health concerns. In E. Youngkin & M. Davis (Eds.), *Women's health: A primary care clinical guide* (3rd ed., pp. 823–860). Upper Saddle River, NJ: Pearson Education.

National Eating Disorders Association. (2002a). *Causes of eating disorders.* Retrieved September 2, 2005, from http://www.nationaleatingdisorders.org/p.asp?WebPage_ID=286&Profile_ID=41144

National Eating Disorders Association. (2002b). *Eating disorders information index.* Retrieved September 2, 2005, from http://www.nationaleatingdisorders.org/p.asp?WebPage_ID=294

Resources

Gurze Books, Eating Disorders Resources: www.bulimia.com
National Association of Anorexia Nervosa and Associated Disorders: www.anad.org
National Eating Disorders Association: www.edap.org; hot line: 800-931-2237
Something Fishy Web site on Eating Disorders: www.something-fishy.org

Chapter 14
Domestic Violence

Janet Akers, MSN, RN, CEN

Background

Abuse is an intentional act that one person uses in a relationship to control the other. For purposes of this chapter, the female is considered the victim and the male the perpetrator. The reverse scenario also may be true.

14.1 What is domestic violence?

Domestic violence is not an accident! It does not happen because someone was stressed, drinking, or using drugs. Domestic violence is not an isolated, individual event. It is a pattern of behaviors, multiple tactics, and repeated events used by one person in a relationship to control the other. Partners may be married or not married; heterosexual, gay, or lesbian; living together, separated, or dating. Violence can be a criminal offense involving physical assault, sexual abuse, and/or stalking. Emotional, psychological, and financial abuse are not criminal behaviors but are forms of abuse and can lead to criminal violence. Domestic violence also is known as "intimate partner violence."

14.2 Domestic violence has been defined as abuse of one household member or family member by another. Who qualifies as a family or household member?

Unless they have a child in common, the victim and the offender generally must live together or previously have lived together to qualify as family or household members. However, laws vary from state to state. It is important for people to be familiar with the laws in the state where they reside.

14.3 What is the cycle of violence?

The cycle of violence is the pattern that domestic violence has been found to follow. Dalpiaz (2004) described three parts to the pattern.

Part one is the buildup of tension. The partner will seem "on edge." Building of anger, blaming, arguing, and strong mental abuse occur. The partner may feel the need to keep the abuser calm. A breakdown of communication occurs during this phase.

Part two begins when the violence erupts. The abuser "blows up," and physical harm starts. Examples of harm are hitting, slapping, kicking, choking, sexual abuse, threatening, and the use of objects or weapons to terrorize or injure the partner.

Part three is the calm or cooling-off stage. The abuser may apologize and promise that the abusive behavior will never happen again. The abuser may deny the violence or excuse it based on drinking or some other behavior. The abuser may blame the victim for causing the abuse or say that it was not as bad as the victim claims. The abuser may act as though it never happened. The abuser may give gifts of flowers, dinner out, or other things valued by the partner in an effort to smooth things over. The victim hopes the abuse is over and that the abuser can be trusted not to do it again. The victim may try to "do better" so as to not cause further abuse. However, without interventions, over time the cycle will start over, and the violence will get worse. The length of time between part three and the start of a new cycle becomes shorter.

Q 14.4   What are common myths about domestic violence?

- Domestic violence is not a problem in this community.
- Domestic violence only happens to the poor or people of color.
- Some people deserve to be hit or abused.
- The causes of domestic violence are alcohol, drug abuse, stress, and mental illness.
- Domestic violence is just a personal problem between a husband and wife.
- If a woman really was being abused, she would just leave.

Risk Factors

Q 14.5   What are the risk factors for domestic violence?

Domestic violence crosses all race, gender, and socioeconomic lines. According to Berry (2000), some common risk factors are poor socioeconomic status (unemployed or low income), age 18–30, drug or alcohol abuse, isolation from family and friends, partners of different religions or cultures, living in the city rather than a rural or suburban area, a household where husbands/male partners control the decision making, and previous involvement with domestic violence (either as victim or perpetrator).

Q 14.6 Are domestic violence and homelessness related?

When women leave abusive relationships, they often have nowhere to go, especially if they have few resources. Because shelters frequently receive more requests for assistance than they can provide, sometimes victims and their children are forced to choose between abuse at home and life on the streets.

Q 14.7 Is domestic violence ever the victim's fault?

Never! No justification exists for violent behavior. Violence against women by anyone is always wrong. It does not matter if the abuser is a current or past spouse, boyfriend or girlfriend, date, family member, friend, or stranger. The victim did not cause the abuse to occur and is not responsible for the violent behavior of someone else.

Q 14.8 Does the risk for violence against women change with age? Pregnancy? Income?

Violence does not discriminate and is found among all ages, economic situations, educational backgrounds, and racial backgrounds. However, some women may be at greater risk than others. Women with incomes under the poverty level are more likely to become victims than women with higher incomes.

Some studies suggest that 25%–35% of all women who are battered are battered during pregnancy (Berry, 2000). Physical violence may start or increase in severity during pregnancy. The physical abuse may lead to miscarriage and increases the risk of delivering a low-birthweight infant.

Violence against women can occur at any age and includes child abuse and elder abuse.

Q 14.9 What can I do if someone is threatening or abusing me?

Call 911 for help! Women should use the safety plan they have developed (see Question 14.21). Seek safe shelter. Report the abuse, and take legal action immediately. File a criminal and/or a civil protection order as soon as possible. Abused women can call a domestic violence program in their area or call the National Domestic Violence Hotline at 800-799-SAFE (7233) or their state domestic violence hot line. If the woman's employer has an employee assistance program, she should call for assistance. This is a confidential, accessible resource that can provide immediate help and support.

Other resources that are available to help abused women include local churches, hospitals, urgent care centers, and healthcare providers.

Q 14.10   How do I recognize if someone is involved in an abusive relationship?

A woman's behavior at work sometimes may offer clues as to whether she is being abused at home. Chronic absenteeism, preoccupation, and deteriorating job performance may be indicators. She may have a habit of wearing inappropriate clothing, such as long-sleeved clothing in hot weather. Perhaps she is obsessed with arriving and leaving the workplace, school, or store at the same time each day. Heightened anxiety or refusal to alter times, such as come early or stay late, may be an indication that the abuser is expecting her to be at a specific place at a specific time.

Q 14.11   What can I do if I think someone is involved in an abusive relationship?

The most important thing others can do is to express their concern to her. However, she may not acknowledge she has a problem and may lash out at those trying to help. People should not expect an answer but should let her know that they and others are available to help her to find the resources she needs. She should not be expected to leave the relationship immediately. This may not be the best time for her to do so. People should continue to restate their concerns and let her know they are available to help.

Signs/Symptoms

Q 14.12   What are the characteristics of abusers?

No "typical" abuser exists, and an abuser is not easy to spot. In public, abusers may appear friendly and loving to the partner and/or family. Frequently, the abuse occurs behind closed doors. Abusers may try to hide the abuse by causing injuries that can be hidden and/or do not need medical attention.

Abusers often have low self-esteem. They do not take responsibility for their actions. They may even blame the victim for causing the violence. In most cases, men abuse female victims, but it is important to remember that women also can be abusers, and men can be victims.

Q 14.13   What are the characteristics of abuse victims?

Anyone can become a victim of domestic violence. Victims can be any age, sex, race, culture, religion, educational level, employment status, or marital status. Most victims are women, but men also can be victims of domestic or partner violence. Children in homes where domestic violence occurs are more likely to be abused or neglected. Children who are not physically harmed still may have emotional and behavior problems as a result of witnessing domestic violence.

Q 14.14   How do I know if I am abused?

If a woman thinks she might be abused, she should ask herself the following questions. If she answers yes to any of them, she should consider seeking assistance.
- Do arguments with my partner end up with me or someone else being physically hurt?
- Do I avoid my partner's anger to keep from making things worse?
- Do I have to ask permission to do things?
- When my partner calls me stupid, crazy, or weak, am I starting to believe it?
- Have I been made to have sex when I did not want to?
- Have I been made to engage in a type of sexual activity that I did not want to do?
- Am I prevented from seeing my friends or family?
- Am I prevented from getting a job or an education?
- Do I feel isolated and alone?
- Does my partner take my paycheck?
- Does my partner push, hit, slap, choke, kick, or bite me?
- Does my partner threaten me, my children, family members, or pets?
- Does my partner threaten suicide to get me to do something?
- Does my partner use or threaten to use a weapon against me?

Q 14.15   What kind of documentation should I get from a healthcare provider if I have been abused?

If a woman is physically abused, she must go to the hospital or her doctor as soon as possible. Sometimes she may not even know she is hurt. It may take up to four hours or more for a bruise or mark to appear. Abused women may think the injury is small and unimportant, but it could be a bigger injury than they realize. If a woman is pregnant and she was hit in the abdomen, she needs to tell the doctor. Abuse may hurt the unborn child. Domestic violence advocates are available to help and support victims of abuse; women should ask the medical staff to call one for them.

If a woman has been hit or kicked in the head or fell and hit her head, she could be in danger of a closed head injury. If she has memory loss, dizziness, changes in vision, vomiting, or a headache that will not quit, get medical attention immediately. If she finds a mark or injury after she has left the doctor, she should return and have pictures taken. The pictures may be used in court proceedings or to help her to get a protection order.

A victim's medical record will provide evidence that she has sought care for an injury. Should there be questions later about whether an injury occurred, this document will be essential. The victim should be truthful with healthcare providers about the cause of the injury—the best help can be provided if they have the full picture of how an injury occurred.

Interventions

Q 14.16   If I call the police for help, what should I tell them?

If a woman is in danger from an abuser at any time, she should call 911 or the local police department. Some domestic violence programs or shelters provide victims with a cell phone that is programmed to only call 911. The phone is for use when abused women need to call the police and cannot get to any other phone. When the police arrive, they can protect and help them and, if necessary, help children to leave the home safely.

When the police come, the victim must tell them everything the abuser did that made her call. If she has been hit, she should tell the police how many times and show any marks that are present. Remember, it may take up to four hours or more for a bruise or mark to appear. If the woman finds a mark or injury after the police leave, she should call them to return and take pictures. The pictures may be used in court. If the abuser has broken property, the police should be shown the damage.

The police must make a report saying what happened to the victim. The report can be used in court if the abuser is charged with a crime. The victim should get the officers' names, badge numbers, and the report number. The police report can help the victim get a protection order.

14.17   What are some of the concerns that victims of domestic violence may have regarding reporting?

Victims may fear escalating violence from the abuser if he knows the violence has been reported. Victims may be afraid of being blamed for getting help, especially if assistance is obtained outside one's community. Lesbian, gay, or transgendered persons may be afraid of having others find out about their sexual orientation. Victims may be dependent on the abuser for physical, emotional, and financial care. If the victim is a male, he may be ashamed and/or afraid no one will believe or help him. Victims from foreign countries may be afraid of deportation. Victims with strong religious affiliations may be concerned about the availability of help and feel that there is an expectation they must stay in the relationship and not break up the family.

14.18   What is a personal protection order (PPO)?

A PPO is issued by the court. It is used to protect people from being stalked, battered, threatened, or harassed by another person. PPOs can be obtained by anyone who has been physically, sexually, or emotionally abused by someone they have been married to, lived with, have a child with, or dated. Anyone who has been stalked also can obtain a PPO.

14.19   What precautions should abused women take besides getting a restraining order?

Women should begin to consider leaving their abuser and think of at least four places they could go if they leave their home. Abuse victims also should think about people who might help them if they left and people with whom they could leave money or clothes; they also should think about who might take care of pets. Victims can open a bank account or get a credit card in their name and practice how they could make their departure—for example, take out the trash, walk the pet every day, go to the store. Another precaution is that they need to think about how to take their children safely out of the home. Sometimes women taking their children may put all of their lives in danger. Women need to protect themselves to be able to protect their children. Think about making and reviewing a safety plan (see Question 14.21).

Q 14.20   Why do victims stay in an abusive relationship?

Many reasons exist for why people may not leave. Many people who are being abused do not see themselves as victims, and abusers do not see themselves as abusive. Not leaving does not mean that the situation is okay or that the victim wants to be abused. Leaving can be dangerous. It is the *most* dangerous time for women who are being abused.

Q 14.21   What is a personalized safety plan?

A safety plan can help victims to increase their personal safety. The following suggestions are some things they can do.
- If their abuser still lives in their home, they should
  - Have important phone numbers nearby. Numbers they may need are police hot lines, friends, and the local shelter.
  - Tell a friend or neighbor about the abuse. Ask that individual to call the police if he or she hears angry or violent noises.
  - Teach children how to dial 911. Victims can make up a code word that they can use when they need help and need the children to call 911.
  - Preprogram emergency numbers into the telephone, including 911.
  - Practice how to get out of the home safely, and practice with their children.
  - Know the safest places in a home—where there are exits and no weapons. If victims think abuse is going to happen, they should try to get their abuser to one of these safer places.
  - Try to leave, if possible.
- If the abuser lives elsewhere, victims should (Weiss, 2003)
  - Change the locks.

- Install a security system, smoke alarms, and outside lighting system.
- Preprogram emergency numbers into the telephone, including 911.
- Notify neighbors about any restraining orders or separation orders. Ask them to call police immediately if they see the abuser near the home or hear angry or violent noises.
- Tell those who care for their children about the situation and make sure the caregivers know who has authorization to pick up the children.
- Avoid banks, stores, and other places that they frequented when living with the abuser.
- Notify their work supervisor and try to arrange for their calls to be screened.
- Report any abuse of a restraining order immediately, even if it is seemingly innocuous, such as a telephone call or letter.

Q 14.22   I want to leave my abusing partner. What should I do?

Women should get prepared before leaving. They should keep their purse close to an exit door and carry important papers in their purse or keep them in a safe place (e.g., with a friend or family member, safety deposit box, locked in their desk at work). Women should try to have some money hidden with the papers. Emergency phone numbers should be kept in their purse, with the papers, and close at hand in the house.

Victims preparing to leave should tell someone they trust, a person who will not communicate their plans to the abuser and will support them and help them to leave. The "leaving checklist" (Question 14.25) provides more suggestions.

Remember: Abusers try to control their victims' lives. If an abuser feels a loss of control, such as when a victim tries to leave, the abuse gets worse. Victims need to take special care when leaving and continue being careful even after they have left.

Q 14.23   If I am being abused and decide to leave, where should I go?

Victims may be able to stay with friends or relatives. Victims should enlist their help and their promise not to reveal where they are staying to the abuser or his friends and relatives. A woman should not stay with a man unless he is a relative because living with a man she is not married to could hurt her chances of gaining custody of her children and possible spousal support. Victims may choose to go to a women's shelter. Also, they can always call 911 for help.

Q 14.24   If I leave, should I always take the children with me?

If women can do it safely, then they should definitely take their children with them. It may be more difficult to get them later. If women are in immediate danger and cannot take their children, then they still need to leave. Women must ensure their own safety so that they can protect their children later. After leaving, the woman should get legal custody of them within a few days. This is very important. If women do not have their children with them, it may be hard to file for temporary custody. The parent who has physical possession may have an advantage in getting custody. If a woman was successful in leaving with her children, she must be cautious and alert. The abusive partner may try to kidnap, threaten, or harm the children in order to get the victim to return.

Q 14.25   What is a "leaving checklist"?

A leaving checklist is a list of important papers and other necessary items for routine daily life that victims will need before leaving an abusive relationship. The following list is not in a specific order, nor all-inclusive. If women cannot take the originals of documents, they should try to get copies to take.
- Divorce papers, custody orders, PPOs
- Lease or rental agreement or house deed
- Mortgage payment booklet
- Current unpaid bills
- Insurance papers
- Address book
- Pictures and items of sentimental value
- Children's favorite toys, blankets, and other items
- Identification and Social Security cards
- Birth certificates for themselves and their children
- School records and books
- Medications and medical records
- Money, bank books or blank checks, and credit cards
- Keys for their car, house, and workplace
- Car registration and driver's license
- Change of clothing for themselves and their children
- Welfare or other identification
- Passports, green cards, or work permits

Q 14.26   If I go to a shelter, what could I expect?

When women call 911 or a local shelter, staff will instruct them how to get to the shelter. The shelter's address is kept confidential to prevent the abusive partner from finding the victim. Women may bring their children, and there is no charge for emergency shelter services. Usually other adults and children will be there who are experiencing the same traumas and feelings that the abused woman and her children may be feeling. The main purpose of a shelter is to provide living space away from the abuser.

The staff at the shelter will work with victims to develop an individualized plan of action to free themselves from violence. The first step will be to ensure that the woman and her children are physically all right. If she or the children need medical attention, the staff will help to arrange for a physician to see them. They will provide food and a place to stay, sleep, and feel safe. Shelters provide support services and will help abused women to examine their options—legally, educationally, and career-wise. Some may provide programs for children as well.

The next steps are to empower women to examine available opportunities and begin to make decisions regarding the future. This may include helping women with getting restraining orders, obtaining the services of an attorney, retrieving their possessions, getting safe housing, getting their children in school, getting more education or job skills, and obtaining support and counseling for victims and their children. Each shelter may have specific rules that the staff will share with women when they arrive. But remember, the staff are there to help victims and are experienced in helping people who have been abused.

Q 14.27   How does domestic violence affect children?

Children in homes where domestic violence occurs are trauma victims. The children may develop a sense of insecurity, a concern that if they are not safe at home, then they may not be safe anywhere else. The children frequently develop a feeling of worthlessness and low self-esteem. Children from abusive homes are more likely to abuse drugs and alcohol than those who do not come from abusive homes. Children from abusive homes are likely to become abusive in their own relationships. Children in abusive homes have difficulty with building trusting relationships with others. Guilt also may be a side effect; children may feel that they have caused the problem or that they do not deserve to be treated well.

Young children may not be able to express fear and anger at home but may demonstrate aggressive behavior on the playground and in the classroom. They may act as if they are in a fog or miles away from those around them. Boys may react differently than girls. Boys may be more aggressive, getting into fights or hitting walls. The anger is projected onto another child or adult: It is someone else's fault. Girls may turn the tensions inward, withdraw, or become depressed. Instead of acting out, some children try to be perfect.

Q 14.28   How can I help my children to handle domestic violence–related anxiety?

Children can sense the anxiety and tension in the adults around them and experience feelings of helplessness and lack of control that the stress can bring. Children, however, have little experience to help them place the current situation into perspective. Each child will respond differently to the stress and trauma caused by domestic violence.

Some things that parents can do to help are to comfort and frequently reassure children that the violence is not their fault. Parents should be honest and open about the violence. It is okay to say, "I don't know" to answer a child's question. Parents should reassure children that they will do all they can to protect and keep them safe.

Children should be encouraged to express their feelings through drawing, playing, or talking to parents about feelings and fears. Daily routines should be maintained as much as possible. It will take some time for children to regain a sense of trust.

Q 14.29   Can abusers be cured, or should they be punished?

Many opinions about this issue exist. One approach views domestic abuse as the product of a sexist society that accepts male dominance over women; a woman is a man's property, and it is both men's right and their duty to dominate. The view is that power and control are driving forces behind domestic violence; therefore, abusers are controlling people and do not want to change. This model focuses on the here and now—the abuser must stop the abuse, accept responsibility for his actions, or go to jail.

Another view advocates that violence stems from deep character flaws created by traumatic childhood experiences and stunted character development. This model focuses on helping men to change and thereby stop the violence and improve their relationships with women.

Treatment centers have used both models with varying success. Some treatment centers combine ideas from both models to help men to deal with the traumas that may have caused their low self-esteem and the need to control and dominate a partner, while helping them to accept responsibility for their behaviors.

References

Berry, D.B. (2000). *The domestic violence sourcebook: Everything you need to know* (3rd ed.). Los Angeles: Lowell House.

Dalpiaz, C.M. (2004). *Breaking free, starting over: Parenting in the aftermath of family violence.* Westport, CT: Praeger.

Weiss, E. (2003). *Family and friends' guide to domestic violence: How to listen, talk, and take action when someone you care about is being abused.* Volcano, CA: Volcano Press.

Resources

National Coalition Against Domestic Violence: www.ncadv.org

National Domestic Violence Hotline: 800-799-SAFE (7233); Web site: www.ndvh.org

U.S. Department of Agriculture, Safety, Health and Employee Welfare Division. (n.d.). *Domestic violence awareness handbook.* Retrieved September 8, 2005, from http://www.usda.gov/da/shmd/aware.htm

U.S. Department of Justice, Domestic Violence: www.usdoj.gov/domesticviolence.htm

Chapter 15

Chemical Dependency

Zandra Ohri, MA, MS, RN, and Ruth Leslie, RN, CD

Definitions

15.1   What is chemical dependency (also called substance abuse, alcoholism, drug addiction)?

Chemical dependency is a treatable medical disease with certain recognizable signs and symptoms. It is characterized by physical and/or psychological dependence on mood-altering chemicals, denial, tolerance, and relapse. It is a primary disease; that is, it has a definite onset, progression, and conclusion. It is progressive—it gets worse over time. It is chronic. No cure exists, but progression of the disease can be arrested. Finally, it is fatal unless the disease is arrested. (Fatality results from either physical consequences and complications of use or actions taken while under the influence.)

15.2   What is tolerance?

Tolerance is the body's adaptation to mood-altering chemicals. When a woman first consumes the chemical, the cells in her body begin to alter. The more she uses or drinks, the more the body adapts and requires the chemicals in order to "survive." In practice, it means that she must consume more and more in order to get the same effect as the first time or two that the chemicals were used. Unfortunately, the same high never occurs again. Over time, the woman begins to experience withdrawal if she does not get the amount of chemicals her body needs.

15.3   What is relapse?

Relapse occurs when a person who has tried to stay off mood-altering chemicals for a period of time and has tried to work a recovery program begins using drugs or drinking again. Some people are able to work a recovery program (maintain sobriety, carry out the steps of the recovery program, go to meetings, etc.) and never relapse. Some may relapse once and then become convinced that they indeed have a problem. Others, however, have a great deal of difficulty maintaining sobriety. This may be partially because of the degree of illness they are experiencing. For others, lack of support or knowledge may contribute to relapse. In some cases, the reason for lack of ability to maintain sobriety is unknown. Usually the relapse process begins before the person actually begins using or drinking again. The individual starts returning to the former mental state—denying problems, avoiding situations, not working a recovery program, or other issues.

Q 15.4 What is dual diagnosis?

The term "dual diagnosis" is used when a person is both chemically dependent and has a mental health problem. It is not uncommon for women who are chemically dependent to also have a problem with depression. Some people with mental illness actually may use mood-altering chemicals to try to deal with the symptoms of the mental illness. These chemicals could be prescribed medications, over-the-counter drugs, alcohol, or street drugs. Unfortunately, they become addicted to the chemical being used, which then aggravates the mental health problem. Treatment professionals will be unable to determine definitively whether someone has a mental health problem until the mood-altering chemical is removed.

Problem Identification

Q 15.5 What causes people to become chemically dependent?

No specific cause is known. Researchers know that there is a biogenetic trait that is passed along in families; someone in the family has been chemically dependent, such as a parent or grandparent. The person who has this trait metabolizes chemicals differently than most people, and the trait affects the pleasure center in the brain differently. Others may have a problem with mental illness and use mood-altering chemicals to deal with their symptoms. Some who have been sexually abused as children or are currently in abusive relationships will turn to mood-altering chemicals to numb their memories and feelings so that they do not feel the pain of the past and/or current abuse (Becker & Walton-Moss, 2001).

Q 15.6   How many people have a problem with chemical dependency?

The magnitude of the problem is not easy to discern, although it is estimated that 1 in 9–10 people has a problem with chemical dependency. Wide disparities exist in race, ethnicity, and geographic representation; this currently is under study (Community Epidemiology Work Group, 2005).

Q 15.7   How can I tell if a woman is chemically dependent?

The signs and symptoms that a chemically dependent woman displays depend on what chemical(s) is being used, how long she has had a problem, and where she is in her use (actively drinking at that moment, hung over, etc.). In general, deterioration occurs in the person's ability to function in relationships, in the community, and in the job. A chemically dependent person gradually pulls away and focuses all her attention and energy on ensuring that she is getting the chemicals she believes she needs to survive. Her actions are designed to ensure that she gets enough of what she needs when she needs it. She goes from needing a drink or drug to relax or relieve stress, to feeling guilty about her use, and then to believing that other activities are interfering with her drinking or drug use.

In family relationships, the woman may start to withdraw, make excuses, become belligerent, and hide what she is using as well as how much and how often. Finances become strained, and she may end up in severe financial difficulties. She may pull away from the community activities in which she used to participate.

On the job, the woman demonstrates a gradual deterioration and inability to get along with others, an inability to accomplish tasks accurately or in the time frame in which she used to be able to do them, and poor decision making. Her behavior includes increasing absenteeism, coming in late, or leaving early. The employee may experience increasing injuries, illnesses, and hospitalizations (National Institute on Drug Abuse [NIDA], 2004).

Specific signs and symptoms exist according to the substance being used. Please note that chemically dependent people usually use more than one substance at a time, so the signs and symptoms may be confusing or conflicting. Also note that if a person displays one of these symptoms, it does not necessarily mean she is using any particular substance. For example, some people have increased appetite when they are under stress, whereas others lose their appetite. Neither is necessarily an indication of substance abuse. When determining whether a person has a substance abuse problem, one needs to look at the whole picture.

Here are some examples of signs and symptoms according to the chemicals being used.
- **Marijuana** (also known as dope, weed, herb, grass, pot, reefer, Mary Jane): Rapid, loud talking; excessive laughter or inappropriate happiness; forgetfulness in a conversation ("What was I saying?"); inflammation in the whites of the eyes; pupils unlikely to be dilated; appearance of intoxication, but has no smell of alcohol; appearance of sleepiness or stupor in the later stages; distorted sense of time passage and tendency to overestimate time intervals; slowed thinking and reaction time, confusion, and impaired memory and learning; tendency to drive vehicles slowly, below the speed limit; increase in appetite, especially after smoking marijuana; impaired balance and coordination; frequent respiratory infections; increased heart rate, anxiety, and panic attacks; odor similar to burnt rope on clothing or breath; and presence of roach clips (e.g., paper clips, bobby pins, hemostats, tweezers), bongs, or water pipes (NIDA, 2005a).
- **Phencyclidine** (also known as PCP, angel dust, boat, hog, love boat, peace pill): Pupils may appear dilated; mask-like facial appearance; rigid muscles, strange gait; irrational speech or behavior; symptoms of intoxication; hallucinations; violent or frightened reactions; subject to flashbacks; exaggerated physical and mental reactions to situations; disorientation; agitation and violence if exposed to excessive sensory stimulation; and deadened sensory perception (may experience severe injuries while not appearing to notice) (NIDA, 2005e).
- **Amphetamines** (also known as speed, meth, hearts, pep pills, bennies, uppers, peaches, cartwheels, sky-rocket): Dilated pupils; dryness of mucous membranes (dry mouth and lips); excessive sweating and shakiness; reduced or loss of appetite; lack of sleep/insomnia; talkativeness with conversation often lacking continuity, changes subjects rapidly; and unusual energy, accelerated movements, and hyperactivity (NIDA, 2005d).
- **Cocaine** (also known as coke, crack, snow, blow, candy, Charlie, flake, toot, C, bump, rock): Dilated pupils; runny nose, reddened and sore nose, cold or chronic sinus/nasal problems, nosebleeds; respiratory problems; unexplained bursts of energy; restlessness or nervousness; repetitive and nonpurposeful behavior; irritability

and anxiety; long periods without sleeping or eating, likely to be emaciated; increased temperature, chest pain, nausea, abdominal pain, strokes, seizures, headaches; white powder in container and/or around nose; and use or possession of paraphernalia including spoons, razor blades, mirrors, little bottles of white powder, and straws (NIDA, 2005b).

- **Opiates** (also known as horse, smack, junk, H, morpho, dollies, heroin, opium, morphine, codeine, fentanyl, demerol, oxycodone, hydrocodone): Pinpoint pupils that fail to respond to light; respiratory depression; drowsiness; nausea and vomiting; apathy and decreased physical activity; short-lived euphoria or feeling good effects; changes in state of mind, going back and forth from feeling alert to drowsy; coma or death (result of overdose); and staggering gait (heroin) (NIDA, 2005c, 2005f).

- **Alcohol:** More irritable, withdrawn; mood swings; isolated—wants to work alone, lunches alone, avoids informal staff get-togethers; elaborate excuses for behavior such as being late for work; blackouts—complete memory loss of events, conversations, or phone calls to colleagues; euphoric recall of events; job shrinkage—does minimal work necessary; difficulty meeting schedules and deadlines; illogical or sloppy documentation and paper work; increasingly absent with inadequate explanations; long lunch hours, sick leave after days off; calls in to request compensatory time at the beginning of the shift; and change in physical appearance (National Institute on Alcohol Abuse and Alcoholism, 2002).

Additional general evidence of active addiction may include inconsistent stories or not remembering what was said; behaviors that are not "normal" for that person (such as yelling, hitting, vulgar language, lewd behavior, crying, or self-pity on more than one occasion after drinking or taking drugs); drinking more than anyone else on a regular basis; going from doctor to doctor with different ailments related to pain; asking for pain medication; using different pharmacies to get pain medication prescriptions filled; weight loss from not eating because of taking drugs or drinking alcohol; grandiose behaviors; accidents on a regular basis that result in injuries that cause pain; legal problems; abnormal sleeping patterns; avoidance of eye contact; unexplained money loss; financial problems; unexplained bruises; needle marks on arms, hands, legs, toes; personality changes; outright lying; paranoia—everyone is out to get them; isolation; changes in appearance for the worse; depression; mood swings; and feelings of impending doom.

Intervention and Treatment

15.8   What do I do if I suspect someone has a problem?

If the person is a family member, contact a treatment facility in the community or nearby and talk with a chemical dependency treatment counselor. This person can help concerned family members to sort through what is happening and discuss how to deal with the situation and potential consequences. If the treatment facility does not have anyone who can talk with concerned relatives, ask for a referral. Consider seeking assistance from other healthcare professionals or religious leaders who have special training in chemical dependency. Al-Anon also provides support for family members, and Alateen helps teenagers who have a family member with a problem (www.al-anon.alateen.org). It is important to realize that chemically dependent people will not automatically get better. They need assistance. Family members may or may not be able to help. If the chemically dependent person fails to follow through and get help, relatives need to be prepared to focus on the protection and needs of the rest of their family and themselves. It is not their fault if the person fails to become or stay sober.

If the person is a coworker, talk with a supervisor. Document job performance problems as they occur. Write down what happened, when, and where, who was involved or observed the incident, and any follow-up provided. Stick to the facts, and keep personal opinions out of the statement. The employer can do nothing without documentation. Over time, the data will indicate the type of problem the person has, such as a chemical dependency problem, a knowledge deficit problem, or a psychological/mental health problem. The supervisor will be able to take action when there is sufficient evidence. Early detection of this disease is paramount.

If a person suspects his or her supervisor has a problem, it is essential to document job performance problems and then meet with the supervisor's supervisor. It is possible that a person will never know the outcome about a fellow coworker because employers try to maintain the employee's privacy.

15.9   What is an intervention?

An intervention is conducted to help chemically dependent people to stop the use of mood-altering chemicals and get into treatment

(Johnson, 1986). An intervention is an activity that needs to be planned and carried out with professional assistance. The interveners should present facts about the person's behavior in an objective, nonjudgmental, and caring way. The interveners present the person with the choice of going into treatment or experiencing serious consequences if he or she does not go into treatment. These consequences may include loss of a job, referral to a regulatory board if the person has a professional license such as nursing or medicine, or loss of family (including loss of support, child custody, or family relationships). The consequences depend on who is doing the intervention—family or employer. It is essential that each intervener be committed to the process, be prepared with facts about the person's behavior, and be prepared to carry out the consequences if the person refuses to get help. Interveners also need to be aware that the person being confronted may respond with anger, denial, blaming, acting out, or suicidal thoughts. The intervention team must be prepared emotionally and factually and have plans to get the person into treatment immediately. The person should not be left alone after the intervention because of the risk of suicide. More than one person should accompany him or her to the assessment/treatment facility. In addition, after the intervention, the team needs time to decompress and talk about what happened and how they feel about the experience.

Q 15.10   What do I do if the intervention does not work?

If the person refuses to go for assessment or treatment, or goes to treatment and refuses to complete it, interveners need to be prepared to follow through on the consequences presented in the intervention. If the chemically dependent person is told that he or she will be fired, then that needs to occur. If the person is a licensed professional, the regulatory board needs to be informed. If the substance abuser is a spouse or significant other and was told that he or she could not return home or that the partner would leave, then the partner needs to ensure that happens.

Interveners then need to look at how to protect themselves and take care of themselves emotionally. If the person with the chemical dependency is a family member, perhaps speaking with a counselor or going to Al-Anon, a support group for friends and family of alcoholics, will help relatives deal with their feelings of anger, disappointment, or betrayal. Do the relatives need to speak with an attorney or get a restraining order? Do their children need help in coping?

If the person confronted was an employee or coworker, does the unit or department need help dealing with feelings of anger and disappointment? Is there someone in the organization who can assist—a chaplain, counselor, or nurse? Is someone available for other employees to go to and discuss how they are feeling? It is essential that other employees not ignore these feelings. They will not go away by ignoring or denying them.

Q15.11   What does treatment involve?

Several different kinds of treatment are available. Treatment usually depends on what the person's insurance coverage includes (if the person is insured) and what kind of chemicals he or she has used. Treatment may range from detoxification (observation the first few days after stopping all chemicals), to inpatient care, or to outpatient care. Very few insurance plans today cover inpatient care, but many plans cover intensive outpatient programs. Treatment provides physical and emotional assistance to the person coming off the drugs, help in learning about the disease, and assistance in practicing behaviors that will support a recovery program. Usually treatment programs also have an aftercare component that involves meeting with a treatment counselor weekly. Halfway houses and three-quarter-way houses are available for people who need further assistance.

Q15.12   How do I find out what treatment facilities are available in my community?

People can check in the yellow pages under "hospitals" or with their insurance company. Other ways are to ask the employee health service nurse at their job if one is available, contact their employee assistance program, talk with their minister or healthcare provider, or research the topic on the Internet. If they are in a small community, they may need to look in a nearby larger town for a place to get help. Some states have alcohol, drug addiction, and mental health boards that can provide assistance. People also should check whether a prospective treatment facility is certified or approved by a state regulatory board to provide treatment. The treatment facility should be willing to provide this information when asked.

Q15.13   What are 12-step programs?

12-step recovery programs consist of 12 steps that people who participate need to follow. These are totally voluntary programs that have helped millions throughout the world (Alcoholics Anonymous, 2005). Programs are available for alcoholics (Alcoholics Anonymous), drug addicts (Narcotics Anonymous), cocaine addicts (Cocaine Anonymous), and others. Equivalent types of programs for family members and friends are Al-Anon and Alateen. These programs help people to work on sobriety and recovery for the remainder of their lives. They provide support and education regarding how to cope with emotions, sobriety, cravings, relapse, and relationships.

Recovery

15.14   What is recovery?

Recovery is a lifelong process that involves several components. It is not sufficient for chemically dependent people to simply abstain from the use of mood-altering chemicals. They are just "dry" at this point. They first must admit to having a problem and then alter the way information is received, processed, and interpreted. Alcoholics and addicts, when actively using or beginning the relapse process, are focused on doing whatever it takes to keep on using. Nothing else matters. Someone who is working a recovery program must learn how to change focus, how to relate to people and situations, and how to function as an adult. This person also needs to develop emotionally.

A recovery program includes maintaining sobriety (not using mood-altering chemicals), going to 12-step meetings regularly, working with a sponsor in the program, working on the 12 steps of recovery, looking at one's own behaviors and thought patterns and how they need to be changed or improved, helping others, and learning how to work with and relate to other people. It takes a lifetime to accomplish this. One recovering nurse said that she always felt as though everyone else got this "book" that told him or her how to be, feel, and act. She always felt as though she was out of step or the odd man out because she did not get this same book. Her recovery program gave her that "book."

15.15   What happens if the person in recovery is injured or has to have surgery?

Recovering people have the same likelihood of becoming ill or injured as do other people. Just as with non–chemically dependent people, chemically dependent people need adequate pain control. If someone tells a medical professional that he or she is an alcoholic or addict or is in recovery, the first question healthcare providers should ask is, "When was your last drink or drug use (sobriety date)?" Then ask about the chemical dependency history (drug of choice), treatment history, and recovery program. The recovering person is expected to tell each healthcare professional providing treatment about his or her disease. Consider all of these factors in determining how best to treat this client. For example, if the person needs pain medication, the prescription should be limited to the minimum drug, dosage, and time frame that the pain medication is needed. If the person needs more pain medication, he or she should go back to see the prescriber to be reevaluated. No refills should be given on the original prescription. The healthcare provider also should ask the person about his or her sponsor: Has the sponsor been told? When will this happen (if an accident has occurred and the person has not yet had time to make contact)? What extra steps are being taken to maintain sobriety? In addition, help the person to look at some additional actions that can be used to supplement the pain medication. Ice packs, elevation of an affected extremity, relaxation exercises, meditation, and rest are examples of nonpharmacologic interventions. Someone should be available in the home or close to the recovering person to help to manage or monitor the medication use—no matter how long the person has been clean and sober.

Q 15.16   What about nurses or other healthcare providers who are chemically dependent?

Just as in the general population, healthcare providers also may become chemically dependent. Many healthcare providers enter the field because they want to help take care of others. In addition, women often believe that everyone else's needs should come before their own. Women caregivers combine these two potentially volatile characteristics.

Certain characteristics of both society and the healthcare profession also can contribute to the risk of becoming chemically dependent. For example, as a society, Americans believe that in order to deal with a problem, people should take a pill. People do not stop to ask why they have this headache and deal with the cause of the headache. Instead, they pop a couple of pills and keep going. This is called "pharmacologic optimism." Healthcare providers may believe that their knowledge about drugs will protect them from becoming chemically dependent. Their work is very stressful and demanding, and they may have a false belief that they should never get sick like their patients. Healthcare providers have easy access to drugs, either at work or by knowing which physicians to go to and what to complain about physically. One way of dealing with burnout is to take a drink or a pill to relieve their emotional pain. They also may experience post-traumatic stress from being exposed to grief, death, and dying on a daily basis. No one factor causes chemical dependency. The interplay of many factors involving both genetics and personality can create problems.

Q 15.17   What help is available for impaired healthcare professionals?

Help varies based on the healthcare professionals' community and state. Some professional associations (nursing, medicine, pharmacy, dentistry, and others) provide varying kinds of services, including interventions, referrals to treatment facilities, support groups, or monitoring programs. In some states, the regulatory board for a particular discipline may have an organized program. Special support groups may exist in their area. To find out what is available in their state, people seeking help can contact the state professional association first. For nursing, the American Nurses Association provides a listing of all the constituent member associations on its Web site at www.nursingworld.org.

References

Alcoholics Anonymous. (2005). *The recovery program.* Retrieved September 1, 2005, from http://www.aa.org/en_information_aa.cfm?PageID=2&subpage=56

Becker, K., & Walton-Moss, B. (2001). Detecting and addressing alcohol abuse in women. *Nurse Practitioner, 26*(10), 13–16, 19–25.

Community Epidemiology Work Group. (2005, August). *Epidemiologic trends in drug abuse* (NIH Publication No. 05-5280). Retrieved September 1, 2005, from http://www.drugabuse .gov/PDF/CEWG/AdvReport_Vol1_105.pdf

Johnson, V. (1986). *Intervention: How to help someone who doesn't want help.* Minneapolis, MN: Johnson Institute Books.

National Institute on Alcohol Abuse and Alcoholism. (2002). *FAQs on alcohol abuse and alcoholism.* Retrieved September 1, 2005, from http://www.niaaa.nih.gov/FAQs/General-English/

National Institute on Drug Abuse. (2004, December). *Criteria for substance dependence diagnosis.* Retrieved September 1, 2005, from http://www.drugabuse.gov/Drugpages/DSR .html

National Institute on Drug Abuse. (2005a, February). *Marijuana: Facts parents need to know.* Retrieved September 1, 2005, from http://www.nida.nih.gov/MarijBroch/parentpg7-8N .html

National Institute on Drug Abuse. (2005b, March). *NIDA InfoFacts: Crack and cocaine.* Retrieved September 1, 2005, from http://www.nida.nih.gov/infofacts/cocaine.html

National Institute on Drug Abuse. (2005c, March). *NIDA InfoFacts: Heroin.* Retrieved September 1, 2005, from http://www.nida.nih.gov/infofacts/heroin.html

National Institute on Drug Abuse. (2005d, May). *NIDA InfoFacts: Methamphetamine.* Retrieved September 1, 2005, from http://www.drugabuse.gov/infofacts/methamphetamine.html

National Institute on Drug Abuse. (2005e, March). *NIDA InfoFacts: PCP (phencyclidine).* Retrieved September 1, 2005, from http://www.drugabuse.gov/infofacts/pcp.html

National Institute on Drug Abuse. (2005f, February). *NIDA InfoFacts: Prescription pain and other medications.* Retrieved September 1, 2005, from http://www.nida.nih.gov/infofacts/PainMed.html

Resources

Crosby, L., & Bissell, L. (1989). *To care enough: Intervention with chemically dependent colleagues. A guide for healthcare and other professionals.* Minneapolis, MN: Johnson Institute Books.

Hazelden (treatment facility; written and video resources): www.hazelden.org/bookstore

National Clearinghouse for Alcohol and Drug Information: www.health.org

National Institute on Alcohol Abuse and Alcoholism: www.niaaa.nih.gov

National Institute on Drug Abuse: www.nida.nih.gov

Peer Assistance Program for Nurses, The Institue for Nursing: www.njsna.org/practice/peer.html

Chapter 16
Nutrition for Health Promotion

Diana Fullen Bowers, PhD, RD, LD

Weight Management

16.1 What is body mass index, and how is it calculated?

Body mass index (BMI) is an anthropometric measure used to help determine the appropriateness of adult weight for height. Because BMI does not measure body fat, a person with a large muscle mass and lower percentage of body fat may have the same BMI as a person with a lower muscle mass and greater percentage of body fat. For this reason, BMI is one of many measurements that collectively help to determine the risk of chronic disease such as diabetes, heart disease, high blood pressure, osteoarthritis, and some cancers. The formula to calculate BMI is weight ÷ (height)^2, where weight is in kilograms and height is in meters. A BMI less than 18.5 is considered underweight, 18.5–24.9 is considered a normal weight, 25–29.9 is considered overweight, and a BMI greater than 30 indicates obesity (Centers for Disease Control and Prevention, 2005).

16.2 How can I determine my ideal body weight?

Ideal body weight (IBW) typically is calculated using the Hamwi (1964) formula. For women, begin with 100 pounds for the first five feet in height. Then add an additional five pounds for each additional inch. For example, the IBW for a woman who is 5'7" is 100 pounds + (5 x 7) = 135 pounds. A range of plus or minus 10% usually is applied, making a weight of 121.5–148.5 acceptable for a 5'7" woman.

For men, begin with 106 pounds for the first five feet, and then add six pounds for each additional inch. The IBW for a man who is 6'2" is 106 pounds + (6 x 14) = 190 pounds, with a range of 171–209 being acceptable.

Q 16.3 What are the health risks associated with having an increased waist-to-hip ratio ("apple" versus a "pear" shape)?

Body fat distribution appears to play a role in the development of co-morbid conditions associated with obesity. The "apple shape" describes the accumulation of fat above the waist, whereas the "pear shape" refers to fat accumulation in the lower abdomen, buttocks, hips, and thighs. Upper body fat (apple shape) is associated with a greater risk for hypertension, cardiovascular disease, hyperinsulinemia (high blood-sugar levels), diabetes mellitus, gallbladder disease, stroke, and cancers of the breast and endometrium (Pi-Sunyer, 1996). The waist-to-hip ratio is a measurement to determine whether a person has an apple or a pear shape. Women can determine the ratio by dividing their waist measurement by their hip measurement. For women, a number greater than 0.8 has been shown to predict complications from obesity, independent of BMI (Bjorntorp, 1985).

Q 16.4 What is metabolic syndrome, and how is it affected by diet?

Metabolic syndrome, also called syndrome X or insulin-resistance syndrome, is characterized by central obesity (apple shape), high blood pressure, high triglyceride levels, low levels of high-density lipoprotein cholesterol (the good cholesterol), and hyperinsu-linemia (American Heart Association, 2005). People with metabolic syndrome are at a greater risk for heart attack and stroke. Metabolic syndrome is thought to be genetically linked, although the underlying cause is not yet fully understood. Dietary factors that may contribute to the development of metabolic syndrome include an excessive caloric intake and a high saturated fat intake.

Q 16.5 How can I avoid developing metabolic syndrome?

Diet and exercise affect many of the problems that together characterize metabolic syndrome. Although people can do nothing about their predisposition to metabolic syndrome from a genetic standpoint, many lifestyle interventions can help to prevent or delay the onset of metabolic syndrome. These interventions include achieving and maintaining an IBW, eating a low saturated fat diet, increasing physical activity, not smoking, and controlling blood pressure and blood glucose levels.

16.6 **There are so many "diets" on the market today. How can I evaluate them and choose one that is right for me?**

Americans spend more than $30 billion a year on all types of diet programs and products, including diet foods and drinks. When it comes to weight-loss diets, however, no quick and easy solutions exist. That is why they have such a low success rate. Consumers should avoid diets that claim sensational results, using terms such as "effortless," "guaranteed," "miraculous," or "breakthrough." To lose weight safely and keep it off requires commitment and long-term changes in daily eating and exercise habits. Look for programs that offer the expertise of a registered dietitian, incorporate an exercise routine, and provide group and/or one-on-one support. Before spending money on a diet program, consider these questions.

- What are the health risks?
- Does the program have data that prove it actually works?
- Do customers keep the weight off?
- What are the costs for membership, weekly fees, food, supplements, maintenance, and counseling?
- Are costs covered by insurance?
- Is professional supervision provided? What are the professionals' credentials?
- Does the program require special menus of foods, counseling visits, or exercise plans?

Supplements/Nutrients

16.7 **What kind of calcium is best to take?**

The most common types of calcium available today are oyster shell calcium, calcium carbonate, and calcium citrate. Of these, calcium citrate is the most rapidly absorbed. Although calcium citrate products may contain less calcium per serving, this is offset by the fact that the calcium in this form is more soluble and therefore better absorbed. Calcium citrate may be taken with or without food and is the best choice for patients with achlorhydria (absence of hydrochloric acid in the gastric juice).

Calcium carbonate is relatively insoluble, especially at a neutral pH. For best absorption, women should take calcium in this form with a meal. Because of reports of possible contamination with heavy metals, oyster shell calcium generally is not recommended. Choose a calcium supplement that also provides vitamin D, which is necessary for optimal calcium absorption.

16.8   Does the recommended daily intake of calcium change throughout a woman's life span?

Absolutely! High calcium intake is critical during the years between menarche and late adolescence because it plays an important role in the attainment of optimal bone mineral density. Think of it as building up a bank account for later use. Calcium intake recommendations during the middle years are based on studies that determined intakes at which small gains in bone mineral density were achieved (National Osteoporosis Foundation, 2005). The intake recommendation for later years is based on clinical trial data that demonstrated less bone loss with calcium intakes of more than 1,000 mg/day. The current recommended calcium intake for females, according to the National Institutes of Health Office of Dietary Supplements (2005), is 1,300 mg/day for ages 9–18, 1,000 mg/day for ages 19–50, and 1,200 mg/day for ages 51 and older.

16.9   Besides calcium, what other nutrients are important for bone health?

Although dietary calcium is critical for building bone density, other nutrients play an important role in bone health, as well. Healthy bones require phosphorus along with calcium. Phosphorus is found in foods such as breads, cereals, rice, pasta, meat, fish, and poultry.

Vitamin D is required for the efficient absorption of dietary calcium. Most people get enough vitamin D because the skin produces it when exposed to sunlight. However, people confined to the indoors or who live in northern latitudes may be deficient in vitamin D. To ensure an adequate vitamin D intake, choose vitamin D–fortified milk products and other vitamin D–fortified foods such as cereals.

Two nutrients that may weaken bones are dietary sodium and protein. Both increase urinary excretion of calcium. However, when phosphorus is consumed along with protein, it can diminish the negative effect of the protein. Alcohol also negatively affects bone health by inhibiting calcium absorption.

Q 16.10 What should I keep in mind when reading a food label?

Food labels provide a wealth of information. When reading a food label, first identify the serving size and total calories per serving. Next, check the number of fat calories per serving. Comparing the fat calories to total calories per serving provides an easy way to tell if the food fits into a healthy eating plan of approximately 30% of total daily calories coming from fat. Check to see how much of the fat is from saturated fat—the 2005 dietary guidelines recommend that saturated fat contributes no more than 10% of daily calories (U.S. Department of Health and Human Services [DHHS] & U.S. Department of Agriculture [USDA], 2005). Also check the amount of sodium per serving. The 2005 dietary guidelines recommend consuming less than 2,300 mg of sodium per day (DHHS & USDA).

The column on the label that lists "% daily value" is based on a 2,000 calorie per day intake (U.S. Food and Drug Administration, 2004). This can be a bit confusing, especially if someone is trying to limit calories to 1,200–1,600 calories per day. For this reason, many consumers use the "% daily value" data as a guide to determine if a food is low or high in a particular nutrient. Generally speaking, if an individual nutrient in a food product has a daily value of 20% or more, the food is considered "high" in that particular nutrient. Remember, in the case of saturated fat, sodium, and cholesterol, "high" is not better.

Q 16.11 What is the recommended daily intake of fiber?

The suggested daily fiber intake is 20–35 grams per day. Of this, 5–10 grams should come from soluble fiber. Americans typically fall short of this mark, eating approximately 12–17 grams of fiber per day, with 4 grams or less coming from soluble fiber (DHHS & USDA, 2005).

Q 16.12 Is it better to eat soluble or insoluble fiber?

Soluble fiber, found in foods such as oats, peas, beans, and certain fruits, forms a gel when mixed with liquid. Soluble fiber is helpful in managing blood glucose levels and lowering serum cholesterol. The recommendation is for people to include 5–10 grams of soluble fiber in their daily diet (DHHS & USDA, 2005).

Insoluble fiber is the fiber that passes through a person's digestive system basically intact. Insoluble fiber is helpful in the alleviation of some digestive disorders, promotes bowel regularity, and is linked to the prevention of colon cancer. Food sources of insoluble fiber are wheat bran, corn bran, whole-grain breads and cereals, certain vegetables, fruit skins, and nuts.

Q16.13   I usually eat on the go. Are there any "easy" ways to increase my fiber intake?

Many easy ways exist for people to increase their daily fiber intake. Consider choosing whole-grain bread and brown rice; snacking on popcorn, fresh vegetables, dried fruits, or nuts; choosing whole fruits instead of juice, eating fruits and vegetables with the skin on, and choosing the restaurant's vegetarian dish—and do not forget the beans!

Q16.14   What are trans fatty acids? Is it important to avoid them?

Trans fatty acids are unsaturated fatty acids that have been partially hydrogenated by heating the liquid oil in the presence of metal catalysts and hydrogen. The process causes the normally "bent" unsaturated fatty acid, which is liquid at room temperature, to change configuration to a "straight" molecule that is solid at room temperature. This is how vegetable oils are hardened into shortening and margarine. Trans fatty acids are found in the oils used to cook French fries and other fast foods, as well as in commercial baked goods.

The change in configuration from a bent to a straight form causes trans fatty acids to have physiologic properties similar to saturated fatty acids. Trans fatty acids have adverse effects on blood lipid levels (they raise low-density lipoprotein [LDL] or "bad" cholesterol levels) and are associated with an increased risk of coronary heart disease. Based on this evidence, consumers should look for labels that indicate a product is "trans fatty acid free."

Q16.15   What is the relationship between dietary saturated fat and serum cholesterol levels?

Saturated fat has been shown to increase serum cholesterol more than any other dietary factor. It is recommended that less than one-third of a person's daily fat intake (less than 10% of total calories) come from saturated fat. Saturated fat usually is solid at room temperature, and the foods with the highest amounts of saturated fat are animal foods—meat, butter, cream, ice cream, and cheese. Coconut and palm kernel oils also are very high in saturated fat.

Q 16.16   Is there a link between dietary fat intake and breast cancer?

Studies of dietary fat intake and breast cancer risk have produced conflicting results. Some studies show that breast cancer is less common in countries where the diet is low in total fat (15%–20% of total calories), low in polyunsaturated fat, and low in saturated fat. However, other studies show inconsistent results regarding the effects of total fat intake on breast cancer risk (Cornell University Program on Breast Cancer and Environmental Risk Factors in New York State, 1999). Issues such as genetics, activity level, and intake of other nutrients confound possible links between dietary fat and breast cancer.

Recent evidence shows that postmenopausal women who ate a low-fat diet were less likely to develop a recurrence of breast cancer than those who ate a standard diet (National Cancer Institute, 2005). This is the first time a large randomized clinical trial has shown that a low-fat diet can reduce the chance of breast cancer recurrence. Women in the low-fat diet group consumed 20% of their total calories as fat (about 33 grams of fat per day) and experienced a 24% reduction in their risk of recurrence when compared to the standard diet group, who consumed 40% of their total calories as fat (about 51 grams per day). The reduction in breast cancer recurrence cannot be attributed to the low-fat diet with 100% certainty because other factors associated with a low-fat diet, including modest weight loss and increased consumption of fruits and vegetables, also may have contributed to the positive results.

The risk of developing breast cancer is associated with obesity—especially for women after menopause. Fat tissue can change some hormones into estrogen, thereby increasing estrogen levels and the likelihood of developing breast cancer. Women who have gained weight as adults and who have "apple" shapes appear to be at greater risk than women who have been overweight since childhood.

Sound dietary advice is available in *Dietary Guidelines for Americans, 2005* (DHHS & USDA, 2005). These guidelines recommend consuming 25%–30% of total calories from fat, limiting total calories from saturated fat to less than 10%, and keeping trans fatty acid consumption as low as possible. For obese women, even a modest (10%) reduction in weight has health benefits.

Q 16.17   Is it possible to reduce one's blood pressure with dietary intervention?

The Dietary Approaches to Stop Hypertension (DASH) clinical study was designed to determine whether eating a diet of foods high in calcium, potassium, and magnesium could lower blood pressure. The National Institutes of Health (n.d.) funded the study, and the results were published in 1997. The study results showed that a diet low in fat and rich in low-fat dairy foods, fruits, and vegetables could substantially lower blood pressure in people with stage 1 hypertension (blood pressure of 140–159/90–99 mm Hg). The results were equivalent to the effect of using blood pressure medication, and the effects happened within two weeks after starting the diet. The DASH daily intake includes three servings of low-fat milk and dairy foods, four to five servings of fruit, four to five servings of vegetables, seven to eight grain food servings, two or less servings of meat, fish, or poultry, and four to five servings per week of nuts, seeds, and legumes.

Q 16.18   Should I take a daily multivitamin?

A multivitamin should not be used in place of a healthy dietary intake. In fact, experts agree that when consumers make healthful food choices, they receive all of the vitamins and minerals needed for good health. However, in some instances a person will benefit from a daily multivitamin and mineral supplement. These instances may include a diet frequently lacking in the recommended number of servings of fruits and vegetables, a strict vegetarian diet, certain disease states or medical conditions, and very low-calorie weight-loss diets. If people choose to take a multivitamin and mineral supplement, they should select one that provides no more than 100% of the daily value for vitamins and minerals and avoid products that advertise sensational claims on the label.

Q 16.19   I have heard a lot about soy protein and health promotion. What are some of the ways soy promotes health?

Soy foods are good sources of fiber, protein, some B vitamins, and minerals such as calcium and iron. In addition, the isoflavones in soy products are associated with many health benefits. Soy protein has been proved to reduce the risk of heart disease by reducing total cholesterol, LDL cholesterol, and triglycerides, and the isoflavone genistein may prevent the early stages of atherosclerotic plaque. Soy foods help to reduce the risk of osteoporosis by providing dietary calcium, reducing urinary calcium losses, and preventing bone break-down. Some studies have found that soy isoflavones are associated with a reduced risk of breast and prostate cancers and may be helpful in relieving symptoms associated with menopause.

Q 16.20   What does "organic" on a food label mean? Are organic foods better for me?

In October 2002, the USDA put into place a set of national standards that food labeled "organic" must meet, whether it is grown in the United States or other countries. To carry the UDSA organic food seal, products cannot include pesticides or genetically modified ingredients or be irradiated to kill bacteria and lengthen shelf life. Organic foods cannot be produced from animals given antibiotics or growth hormones.

Three types of USDA organic labels exist. Products that are entirely organic will have "100% organic" USDA labels. Those with at least 95% organic ingredients will have a USDA "organic" stamp. Foods with at least 70% organic ingredients cannot use the USDA seal, but their labels can say they are "made with organic ingredients" (National Organic Program, 2002).

Organic food differs from conventionally produced food in the way it is grown, handled, and processed. Organically produced food has not been determined to be safer or more nutritious than conventionally produced food, although some consumers feel that choosing organic products is a simple way to reduce exposure to the potential harm caused by the use of pesticides and fertilizers.

References

American Heart Association. (2005, August). *Metabolic syndrome.* Retrieved August 1, 2005, from http://www.americanheart.org/presenter.jhtml?identifier=4756

Bjorntorp, P. (1985). Regional patterns of fat distribution. *Annals of Internal Medicine, 103,* 994–995.

Centers for Disease Control and Prevention. (2005, August). *BMI—Body mass index: BMI for adults.* Retrieved August 1, 2005, from http://www.cdc.gov/nccdphp/dnpa/bmi/bmi-adult .htm

Cornell University Program on Breast Cancer and Environmental Risk Factors in New York State. (1999, May). *Dietary fat and the risk of breast cancer* (Fact Sheet No. 27). Retrieved September 12, 2005, from http://envirocancer.cornell.edu/factsheet/Diet/fs27.fat.pdf

Hamwi, G. (1964). Changing dietary concepts. In T.S. Danowski (Ed.), *Diabetes mellitus: Diagnosis and treatment* (pp. 73–78). New York: American Diabetes Association.

National Cancer Institute. (2005, May). *Clinical trial results: Low-fat diet may reduce risk of breast cancer relapse.* Retrieved September 12, 2005, from http://www.cancer.gov/clinicaltrials/results/low-fat-diet0505

National Institutes of Health. (n.d.). *The DASH diet.* Retrieved August 1, 2005, from http://www.nih.gov/news/pr/apr97/Dash.htm

National Institutes of Health Office of Dietary Supplements. (2005). *Dietary supplement fact sheet: Calcium.* Retrieved August 1, 2005, from http://ods.od.nih.gov/factsheets/calcium.asp

National Organic Program. (2002, April). *Organic foods standards and labels: The facts.* Retrieved August 1, 2005, from http://www.ams.usda.gov/nop/Consumers/brochure.html

National Osteoporosis Foundation. (2005, August). *Prevention: Calcium supplements.* Retrieved August 1, 2005, from http://www.nof.org/prevention/calcium_supplements.htm

Pi-Sunyer, F.X. (1996). Obesity. In J.C Bennett & F. Plum (Eds.), *Cecil textbook of medicine* (20th ed., pp. 1161–1168). Philadelphia: Saunders.

U.S. Department of Health and Human Services & U.S. Department of Agriculture. (2005, January). *Dietary guidelines for Americans, 2005* (6th ed.). Washington, DC: U.S. Government Printing Office. Retrieved October 20, 2005, from http://www.health.gov/dietaryguidelines/dga2005/document/

U.S. Food and Drug Administration. (2004, November). *How to understand and use the nutrition facts label.* Retrieved August 1, 2005, from http://www.cfsan.fda.gov/~dms/foodlab.html

Resources

American Dietetic Association: www.eatright.org

U.S. Department of Agriculture, National Agricultural Library: www.nutrition.gov

U.S. Food and Drug Administration, Center for Food Safety and Applied Nutrition: www.foodsafety.gov/list.html

Chapter 17

Hormone Replacement Therapy

Janis A. Cruce, MSN, RN, CS, FNP

Background

Q 17.1 What is perimenopause? What is menopause?

Perimenopause officially means the time "around" menopause and begins when a woman's ovaries start to produce fewer hormones. Menopause is medically defined in a woman who has not had a menstrual cycle for one year.

Q 17.2 Should I start taking hormones? Are they safe?

Hormones currently are not routinely used in "treatment" of menopause. Women should discuss hormone replacement therapy (HRT) or hormone therapy with their healthcare provider to find out whether it is right for them. Many women find that severe hot flashes and night sweats during perimenopause prompt their first inquires about hormones.

Q 17.3 Can I take estrogen alone or progesterone alone?

If hormones are prescribed, the women's healthcare provider will keep certain considerations in mind. At times, women may take estrogen or progestin (Provera®, Pfizer Inc., New York, NY) alone or in combination, but always under the care of their healthcare provider. It is only safe for women to take estrogen alone if they no longer have a uterus.

Side Effects

Q 17.4 Can hormones make you fat?

Estrogen can cause water retention. Provera can cause some women to gain a few pounds. A healthy lifestyle with a balance of exercise and healthy eating can help to maintain weight during the peri-menopausal period.

17.5 Can hormones cause breast cancer, stroke, and heart disease?

Recent studies described by the Women's Health Initiative (WHI) (Rossouw et al., 2002) have shown a higher risk of breast cancer, stroke, and heart disease in women who take both estrogen and Provera in certain dosage combinations. Further research is under way.

17.6 What are the risks discovered by the WHI study?

Risks discovered by the WHI study (Rossouw et al., 2002) are that during one year, for every 10,000 women taking estrogen plus progestin in the studied dosage combination, healthcare professionals would expect 7 more women with heart attacks, 8 more women with strokes, 8 more women with breast cancer, and 18 more women with blood clots.

17.7 What were the benefits discovered by the WHI study?

WHI study data (Rossouw et al., 2002) suggested that for every 10,000 women taking estrogen plus progestin in the studied dosage combination, healthcare professionals would expect six fewer colorectal cancers, five fewer hip fractures, and fewer fractures in other bones.

17.8 I thought HRT was cardioprotective, and that is why I am taking the pills. Should I continue?

HRT is not protective of a woman's heart and should not be used for that purpose.

17.9 Should I continue HRT if I am at risk for osteoporosis?

If women are at risk for osteoporosis, they should receive treatment with medication that is specifically for osteoporosis. They should consult their healthcare provider regarding options that currently are available.

Nonhormonal Interventions

17.10 What should I do for hot flashes and night sweats?

Other medications are available that can help to decrease hot flashes and night sweats. Clonidine (Catapres®, Boehringer Ingelheim,

Ridgefield, CT) and propranolol (Inderal®, Wyeth, Philadelphia, PA) are antihypertensives that have been found to relieve some of these symptoms. Antidepressants called selective serotonin reuptake inhibitors have been used in patients with breast cancer who suffer from hot flashes and are now being used for other women, as well (Menopause Online, n.d.). Helpful nonpharmacologic actions include avoiding hot beverages and wearing light layers of clothing.

17.11   Will HRT cure my depression?

Hormone replacement is not a cure for depression. If women suffer from depression, they must be evaluated and treated for depression. Hormones play a part in women's moods. Some people feel better when taking hormones, but HRT is not a replacement for treatment of depression.

17.12   How long is it safe to take HRT?

It is very important that women check with their healthcare provider to monitor the need to take and/or continue HRT. Their provider can let them know of the latest findings and recommendations.

17.13   What is the best way to discontinue HRT?

HRT can be discontinued gradually or suddenly. Most healthcare providers support gradual discontinuation.

17.14   What are my alternatives if I want to stop HRT, but my menopausal symptoms are not controlled?

Alternatives include certain blood pressure medications or antidepressants. Some people believe herbal remedies are helpful. A balance of exercise and rest may help. If a woman's quality of life is affected, she needs to consult her healthcare provider and see whether HRT for a short period of time would be helpful. Remember that choices exist. A well-informed woman can make a good choice based on knowing the risks and benefits of treatment methods available.

17.15   What about all these herbal supplements? Are they safe and effective?

The U.S. Food and Drug Administration does not regulate herbal substances. Anecdotal evidence suggests that some people find value in some herbal supplements. However, people must exercise caution in the use of these substances. Be aware of potential side effects or contraindications when taking other prescription or over-the-counter medications.

Q 17.16   What can soy products do for me?

Some women claim that phytoestrogens (or plant estrogens, such as soy) help to relieve menopausal symptoms. No clear evidence exists, however, that soy products are significantly helpful.

References

Menopause Online. (n.d.). *Prescription drugs.* Retrieved September 2, 2005, from http://www.menopause-online.com/drugs.htm

Rossouw, J.E., Anderson, G.L., Prentice, R.L., LaCroix, A.Z., Kooperberg, C., Stefanick, M.L., et al. (2002). Risks and benefits of estrogen plus progestin in healthy postmenopausal women: Principal results from the Women's Health Initiative randomized controlled trial. *JAMA, 288,* 321–333.

Resources

American College of Obstetricians and Gynecologists: www.acog.org

Association for Women's Health, Obstetric and Neonatal Nurses: www.awhonn.org

National Women's Health Information Center, U.S. Department of Health and Human Services Office on Women's Health: www.4woman.gov

Women's Health Initiative: www.whi.org

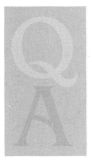

Chapter 18

Herbals and Botanicals

Diana Fullen Bowers, PhD, RD, LD

Background

Q 18.1 **What is the Dietary Supplement Health and Education Act (DSHEA), and what does it mandate?**

The DSHEA is an act passed by Congress in 1994 that amended the Federal Food, Drug, and Cosmetic Act (National Institutes of Health Office of Dietary Supplements [NIHODS], 2004). Prior to passing the DSHEA, dietary supplements were subject to the same regulatory requirements as were other foods. With the DSHEA, however, a new regulatory framework for the safety and labeling of dietary supplements was created.

Under the DSHEA, *manufacturers,* rather than the U.S. Food and Drug Administration (FDA), are responsible for determining that their products are safe and that any claims made about the products are substantiated by adequate evidence to show that they are not false or misleading. The act basically focuses on regulating the marketing and sale of products rather than their safety and effectiveness. The act also

- Defines what a supplement is and what products fall into the supplement category
- Mandates the requirement of a supplement facts label
- Enables the FDA to restrict amounts of potentially dangerous botanicals included in supplements.

Q 18.2 **What is the FDA's role in regulating dietary/herbal supplements?**

Currently, the FDA's role in regulating dietary or herbal supplements is very limited. Manufacturers do not need approval from the FDA before they market a supplement, unless the supplement contains a new dietary ingredient. It is the manufacturer's responsibility to determine this. Furthermore, manufacturers do not have to provide the FDA with evidence of safety or effectiveness before or after a product is marketed. The government cannot restrict the sale of a product unless it can prove the product is unsafe when used according to package directions.

The FDA has proposed a rule to establish manufacturing and labeling standards for all dietary supplements (NIHODS, 2004). These standards will ensure that dietary supplements and dietary ingredients are not adulterated with contaminants or impurities and that they are labeled to accurately reflect the active ingredients and other ingredients in the product.

18.3   Are herbal supplements the same as botanical supplements?

Although people often use the terms "herbal" and "botanical" interchangeably, they are not synonymous. The term "botanical" covers all plants and often refers to vegetable drugs, especially in the crude state. The term "herbal" refers to a small group of plants valued for their medicinal, savory, or aromatic qualities.

18.4   What information must the manufacturer disclose on the label of an herbal supplement?

Herbal supplement labeling requirements went into effect in 1999 (FDA Center for Food Safety and Applied Nutrition, 2001). The label on supplements must include the following information.
- A descriptive name of the product stating that it is a "supplement"
- The name and place of business of the manufacturer, packer, or distributor
- A complete list of ingredients
- The net contents of the product

In addition, the label must include a "supplement facts" panel that identifies the plant botanical name, parts of the plant used, a complete ingredient list, directions for use, and the recommended serving size.

18.5   Why would a person choose to use an herbal supplement?

An estimated 30%–50% of Americans have used or currently are using herbal supplements. Some of the most common reasons people say they use herbal supplements include that herbals are more effective than prescription drugs, herbals have fewer side effects, herbals are safer than prescription drugs, herbals are "natural," use of herbals is consumer controlled and no prescription is needed, and, finally, herbals are used out of frustration when nothing else helps a particular condition.

18.6   What techniques are used in the preparation of herbal products?

Techniques used in the production of herbal products include drying, grinding, extraction, and concentration. Drying reduces the moisture content from 60%–80% to less than 14%. Drying is done to prevent the breakdown of important compounds and to limit contamination by microorganisms. Grinding or mincing is the mechanical breakdown of the whole plant or parts of the plant (leaves, roots, berries, etc.) to a fine powder. Grinding is used in the preparation of crude herbal products and also is the first step in the preparation of an herbal extract. Extraction is the separation by chemical or physical means of the active plant compounds from the parent material using a solvent such as an alcohol and water mixture. The extraction process is used to make tinctures, fluid extracts, and solid extracts. Concentration involves the complete removal of a solvent after the extraction process is complete. Concentration results in a pure fluid or solid extract product.

18.7   How can I be certain that a bottle of ginseng capsules actually contains ginseng?

Supplement manufacturers are responsible for ensuring that the supplement facts label and ingredient list are accurate and that the ingredient amounts declared on the label match those in the product. Currently, no government oversight of this exists. However, an increase has occurred in manufacturer self-regulation and voluntary adoption of "good manufacturing practices" (GMPs) similar to those required by the government for the food and pharmaceutical industries. In addition to choosing products made by manufacturers who voluntarily adhere to industry GMPs, consumers can verify the quality of products through independent companies that test herbal products for quality. These companies include the National Nutritional Foods Association (www.nnfa.org), U.S. Pharmacopeia (USP, www.usp.org), and ConsumerLab.com (www.consumerlab.com).

Q 18.8   How should I choose which part of the plant to use (stem, roots, leaves, berries, or flowers)?

The active ingredient in an herbal product often is concentrated in a certain part of the plant. For example, the active ingredient in saw palmetto is found in the ripe fruit. Therefore, using a tea of saw palmetto leaves will be of little or no benefit. Likewise, the applicable part of the plant feverfew is the leaf—using feverfew root would be of little or no benefit. Before choosing an herbal product, consumers should consult a reliable resource that provides information on the medical prescription of herbs to determine which part of the plant contains the active ingredient indicated for a particular condition.

Q 18.9   Is it better to get an herbal tea, tincture, fluid extract, or solid extract?

The type of product selected depends on which part of the plant contains the active ingredient *and* the solubility of the active ingredient. For example, if the active ingredient is water soluble and is found in the leaf of the plant, then a leaf tea is acceptable. However, if the active ingredient is not water soluble, then a tincture, fluid extract, or solid extract made from the part of the plant containing the active ingredient should be selected.

Q 18.10   Can herbal supplements change the absorption and function of other drugs?

Yes, herbal supplements can change the absorption and function of other drugs. They can diminish or enhance prescription drug absorption and activity, thereby making the prescription drug more or less bioavailable and/or active. Likewise, the prescription drug can diminish or enhance the herbal supplement's absorption and activity. Simultaneous use of an herbal supplement and prescription drug also may produce enhanced potency of both, perhaps leading to undesirable results.

Q 18.11   Because herbal supplements are "natural," aren't they less likely than synthetic drugs to cause side effects?

Many people believe that because herbal products are "natural," their use is less likely to cause adverse side effects. This simply is not true. Many plants found in nature are, in fact, poisonous. Also, because of normal variations in plant components, side effects caused by herbal products may be unpredictable. Keep in mind that if a product has the potential to have a positive effect, it also has the potential to do harm.

Q 18.12   What does "standardization" mean?

"Standardization" means that a supplement has been tested and shown to contain a certain amount of what is thought to be the active ingredient of the parent plant. In other words, the product is standardized to the amount of the active ingredient rather than simply providing a certain milligram or gram weight of the plant product. Standardization, however, does not guarantee that a product is potent or effective.

Q 18.13   Is the actual content of an herbal supplement routinely analyzed?

Manufacturers who adhere to GMPs routinely may analyze their products for standardization and purity. This is not required by law, however, and is not monitored by the FDA. Independent companies do routine analyses of various herbal supplements and make their results available to the public, sometimes for a small fee. ConsumerLab.com is an example of one such company.

Q 18.14   How are advertisements for herbal supplements regulated?

The Federal Trade Commission (FTC) regulates advertisements for herbal supplements. The FDA works closely with the FTC in this area, but the laws governing the FTC are different from those that govern the FDA. The DSHEA mandates that any claims made about herbal supplements be substantiated by adequate evidence to show they are not false or misleading.

Q 18.15   Do herbal supplements have "active ingredients"?

Herbal supplements may contain one or more active ingredients. An active ingredient is a compound that has been shown to be effective in treating or relieving symptoms of a particular condition. Many supplements now are standardized to provide a certain amount of active ingredient per serving. Herbal products may have significant variation in active ingredients based on the brand of supplement, the time of plant harvest, the plant growing conditions, including the climate and soil, and the storage and manufacturing conditions.

18.16   When choosing an herbal supplement, what should I look for on the label?

Consumers can increase the likelihood that they are buying a quality product by checking the label for key information. First, look for a nationally known manufacturer that adheres to GMPs. Look for products that have recognized symbols of quality on the label, such as the USP or NF (National Formulary) insignia. Avoid foreign products and those that make sensational claims. Choose a product that has been standardized, for which the label clearly indicates the quantity of active ingredients. Choose a product that has an expiration date and batch control number, if possible. Finally, check the label for a toll-free customer service telephone number. This helps to ensure that the manufacturer is willing to stand behind the product.

18.17   What is a structure-function claim?

A structure-function claim is a statement that refers to a supplement's effect on the organs or systems of the body, including its overall effect on a person's well-being. This claim cannot mention any specific disease. An example of a structure-function claim is if it "helps support a healthy immune system." Structure-function claims are easy to find on a supplement label because they must be accompanied by the disclaimer, "This statement has not been evaluated by the Food and Drug Administration. This product is not intended to diagnose, treat, cure, or prevent any disease" (NIHODS, 2004).

18.18   What is an adaptogen?

An adaptogen is a substance that is considered safe, increases resistance to stress, and has a balancing effect on body functions. Ginseng is a commonly used adaptogen. It is thought to produce a general stimulatory effect during stress, a decrease in sensitivity to stress, and an increase in mental and physical capacity for work.

Side Effects/Safety

18.19   Can herbal supplements affect the outcome of laboratory tests?

More than 200 different herbal supplements can alter the results of laboratory tests. Some supplements actually can cause the problems detected by the tests, whereas others interfere with test results. For example, liver function tests can be elevated by the use of kava, goldenseal, and red yeast, to name a few. Consumers should thoroughly research any possible interactions between herbal supplements and laboratory tests before beginning supplement use.

Q18.20 **I've heard that black cohosh really works for menopause symptoms. Is it safe to use?**

In some studies, extracts of black cohosh *(Cimicifuga racemosa)* reduced the symptoms of hot flashes, depression, vaginal atrophy, and dysmenorrhea (American Botanical Council, 2005). Remifemin® (GlaxoSmithKline, Research Triangle Park, NC) is the brand name of the standardized extract of the plant. Black cohosh typically is given in the form of a 40%–60% alcohol extract, in a quantity equivalent to 40 mg daily. It may take up to four weeks before maximum beneficial effects are seen.

Although healthcare professionals generally consider black cohosh safe to use, side effects may include nausea, dizziness, nervous system and visual disturbances, reduced pulse rate, and increased perspiration. Studies evaluating the risks of long-term use and toxicity have not been done. Therefore, it is recommended that the use of black cohosh be limited to a period of no longer than six months.

Q18.21 **What other supplements are recommended to relieve symptoms of menopause?**

Phytoestrogens are plant-based compounds that exert a weak estrogenic effect. Commonly found in soy products, phytoestrogens are gaining in popularity as an alternative to hormone replacement therapy in postmenopausal women. Along with soy products, the herbal supplements chaste tree berry *(Vitex agnus-castus),* angelica or Dong quai *(Angelica sinensis),* and licorice root *(Glycyrrhiza glabra)* contain phytoestrogens that some believe to be helpful in relieving symptoms of menopause.

Q18.22 **I have heard a lot about a supplement called "ma huang." What is it, and is it safe to use?**

"Ma huang" is a common name for the many plants of the genus *Ephedra. Ephedra* extracts have a long history of use as stimulants and for the management of bronchial disorders. Many dietary supplements, particularly those touted for weight loss and athletic performance enhancement, include varying amounts of ephedra. Although ephedra technically meets the definition of a botanical regulated under the DSHEA, the principal active alkaloid in the plant is ephedrine, and synthetic ephedrine is regulated as a drug.

Recently, evidence has come to light of potentially serious adverse events following the use of ephedra-containing products. Moderate adverse side effects include gastrointestinal, psychiatric, and autonomic symptoms. Severe adverse side effects with the use of ephedra-containing products may include acute myocardial infarction, stroke, and death. In February 2003, the U.S. Department of Health and Human Services announced a number of actions to address concerns about the safety of ephedra. Because serious adverse events and death were reported after using ephedra, the FDA (2004) banned the sale of dietary supplements containing ephedrine alkaloids on April 12, 2004.

18.23   Why are products containing kava associated with liver damage?

Supplements containing the herbal ingredient kava *(Piper methysticum)* are promoted for the treatment of anxiety, sleeplessness, stress, premenstrual syndrome, and menopausal symptoms. Kava supplements contain a mixture of components collectively known as kava pyrones (i.e., kavalactones). Kava-containing products have been associated with hepatitis, cirrhosis, and liver failure (National Center for Complementary and Alternative Medicine [NCCAM], 2002). Currently, it is not known which compounds in kava cause liver damage, and kavalactones have not been ruled out. On the other hand, it is possible that unknown or unexpected contaminants have contributed to the reported liver toxicity. In March 2002, the FDA released a consumer advisory concerning the association of kava-containing dietary supplements with severe liver injury (NCCAM, 2002).

18.24   How does echinacea help to promote a healthy immune system?

As a general immune stimulant, echinacea increases phagocytosis and serum leukocytes. It also stimulates granulocyte migration and cytokine production. In mice, it is associated with protective effects on influenza A virus infection. Studies to date in humans do not support that echinacea prevents or shortens the course of colds or flu (NCCAM, 2006). The exact compounds responsible for the therapeutic value of echinacea are not known, and commercially available echinacea preparations may be made from several plant species and plant parts. For this reason, it is important to note the source and type of preparation used. People should limit their use of echinacea preparations to eight weeks (American Botanical Council, 2003).

Q 18.25   Are there any side effects associated with the use of St. John's wort?

Some people who have mild to moderate depression use St. John's wort *(Hypericum perforatum)*. Its use is associated with gastrointestinal symptoms, fatigue, delayed hypersensitivity, photosensitivity, and neuropathy. Reports exist of significant drug interactions between St. John's wort and a protease inhibitor used to treat HIV infection. St. John's wort can substantially decrease protease inhibitor plasma concentrations and possibly interfere with the action of other drugs that are metabolized via the cytochrome P450 metabolic pathway (Lumpkin & Alpert, 2000).

Hypericin, the active ingredient in St. John's wort, also is reported to inhibit monoamine oxidase (MAO). People using St. John's wort should avoid foods (such as wines, aged cheese, and chocolates) and medications that are known to interact negatively with MAO-inhibiting drugs. To avoid gastric upset, St. John's wort should be taken with food.

Q 18.26   Can ginkgo really improve memory and circulation?

Some studies show that ginkgo biloba modestly improves memory in some patients with Alzheimer disease, and it might help some patients with other forms of dementia. However, recent evidence shows that it does not improve memory in healthy people older than age 60 (ConsumerLab.com, 2003). As for circulation, some people who have peripheral arterial occlusive disease and tinnitus of vascular origin use ginkgo. Plant ginkgolides improve circulation by inhibiting the binding of platelet-activating factor to its membrane receptor, thereby attenuating platelet aggregation. Because ginkgo teas do not contain enough of the active compounds for therapeutic effects, standardized *Ginkgo biloba* extracts typically are recommended.

Q 18.27   What recourse do I have if I suffer an adverse reaction from an herbal supplement?

If people experience an adverse side effect or reaction while taking an herbal supplement, they should stop taking the supplement immediately. They should report the symptoms to their physician, the product manufacturer, and the FDA. Remember, the government cannot restrict the sale of a product unless it can prove it is unsafe when used according to package directions.

Q 18.28   Do culinary herbs have as many beneficial effects as medicinal herbs?

In addition to enhancing the flavor and presentation of any dish, culinary herbs also provide beneficial phytochemicals such as anti-oxidants, essential fatty acids, and flavonoids. Although the amounts of culinary versus medicinal herbs that one consumes may be very different, keep in mind that culinary herbs offer flavor as well as beneficial phytochemicals.

References

American Botanical Council. (2003). Clinical overview: Echinacea. In M. Blumenthal (Ed.), *The ABC clinical guide to herbs* (pp. 85–96). Austin, TX: Author.

American Botanical Council. (2005, May). *Research on black cohosh supports benefits in menopause.* Retrieved August 2, 2005, from http://www.herbalgram.org/default.asp?c=menopauseupdate

ConsumerLab.com. (2003, April). *Product review: Ginkgo biloba and huperzine A—memory enhancers.* Retrieved August 2, 2005, from http://www.consumerlab.com/results/ginkgobiloba.asp

Lumpkin, M.M., & Alpert, S. (2000, February). *FDA public health advisory: Risk of drug interactions with St. John's Wort and indinavir and other drugs.* Retrieved August 2, 2005, from http://www.fda.gov/cder/drug/advisory/stjwort.htm

National Center for Complementary and Alternative Medicine. (2002, July). *Kava linked to liver damage.* Retrieved August 2, 2005, from http://nccam.nih.gov/health/alerts/kava

National Center for Complementary and Alternative Medicine. (2006, March). *Herbs at a glance: Echinacea.* Retrieved April 8, 2006, from http://nccam.nih.gov/health/echinacea/

National Institutes of Health Office of Dietary Supplements. (2004, July). *Dietary supplements: Background information.* Retrieved August 2, 2005, from http://ods.od.nih.gov/factsheets/dietarysupplements.asp

U.S. Food and Drug Administration. (2004, April). *FDA statement: FDA announces rule prohibiting sale of dietary supplements containing ephedrine alkaloids effective April 12.* Retrieved August 2, 2005, from http://www.fda.gov/bbs/topics/NEWS/2004/NEW01050.html

U.S. Food and Drug Administration Center for Food Safety and Applied Nutrition. (2001, January). *Dietary supplements: Overview.* Retrieved August 2, 2005, from http://www.cfsan.fda.gov/~dms/supplmnt.html

Resources

Consumer Lab.com—Independent tests of herbal, vitamin, and mineral supplements: www.consumerLab.com

Memorial Sloan-Kettering—About Herbs, Botanicals and Other Products: www.mskcc.org/mskcc/html/11570.cfm

National Center for Complementary and Alternative Medicine, National Institutes of Health: http://nccam.nih.gov

Chapter 19
Naturopathic Care

Carolen Koleszar, BSN, RN

Background

Q 19.1 **What is naturopathic care?**

Naturopathic care is an approach to health following the philosophy and practice of naturopathic medicine. The basic principles of naturopathic medicine are to "first, do no harm," to trust in the healing power of nature, and to use various natural methods for healing. A person may receive naturopathic care from anyone educated in this approach. This might include a medical doctor, a chiropractor, or a nurse. Most commonly, one receives naturopathic care from a naturopathic doctor (ND), also known as a naturopath, or a naturopathic medical doctor.

The roots of naturopathic medicine are in Germany, where natural medicine commonly is used and naturopaths are primary care providers. More than 100 years ago, Father Sebastian Kneipp commissioned Dr. Benedict Lust to bring *Nature Cure* teachings from Germany to America (Wood, 2000). This was the beginning of naturopathic medicine in America. Originally, naturopaths were medical doctors who were dissatisfied with the practice of medicine in their day and looked for nonpharmacologic ways to care for their patients. Naturopaths today still believe that disease is a manifestation of an imbalance in the body that occurs when something is lacking (e.g., malnutrition) or when an accumulation of toxins occurs in the body. The goal of the naturopath is to help to remove any obstacles to cure (such as toxicity, malnutrition, or emotional issues) in order to allow nature to do the healing. Healing is facilitated by using natural methods, which include herbal therapy, nutrition, and lifestyle modifications.

Q 19.2   What benefit can I hope to gain from naturopathic care?

Naturopathic care is for improvement in overall health and not necessarily for specific medical conditions. People do not need a medical
diagnosis to benefit from naturopathic care. However, many people
find that their medical conditions improve as they raise their level
of health in general. Under the care of a naturopath, people can
expect to learn about the important basic functions of their body
(such as digestion, elimination, and blood-sugar handling) and how
their health is affected by disturbances in these basic functions.

With naturopathic care, people notice they have more energy, better digestion and elimination, less reliance on stimulants such as
coffee and sugar, and an improvement in overall health. As with
other types of health care, more women than men tend to seek the
services of naturopaths. Naturopaths are experienced in helping
women in particular with a variety of health concerns, especially with
hormonal balance, weight management, and fatigue. As a profession, naturopaths are better known for helping people with natural
medicine in other parts of the world, such as Europe and Australia,
than in the United States.

**Q 19.3   If naturopathic care is so helpful to people in other countries, why
isn't naturopathic care more available here?**

Several reasons exist for this. First, many people are satisfied with the
care they receive from their medical doctors and do not seek an additional healthcare provider. Some people are skeptical about natural
medicine and are not interested in naturopathic care. Other people
might be interested in naturopathic care but are not aware that naturopaths exist or find it difficult or inconvenient to travel to find one.

Also, the licensing issue is a problem for many naturopaths across the
United States. As many states do not offer licensure to naturopaths,
naturopaths are difficult to find in those states. In states without licensure for naturopaths, naturopaths have been arrested and charged
with practicing medicine or chiropractic without a license.

Q 19.4   Is naturopathic care good for everyone?

Not everyone is suited for naturopathic care. This approach requires
a commitment to take responsibility for personal health and make the
effort to change behavior (diet, exercise, and stress management).

Not everyone is willing to make the lifestyle changes that are necessary to improve health through natural methods. This approach is not a "quick fix." Nature does its own healing at its own pace. Healing requires time and the proper conditions.

Naturopathic Practitioners

Q 19.5   How can I find a naturopath?

A naturopath may be listed in the phone book or on the Internet under the heading of "naturopath." Naturopaths also may be found under the heading "holistic practitioners" or "alternative medicine." Health food store staff may be familiar with naturopaths in the area. Most often, people find naturopaths through friends or family by word of mouth.

Q 19.6   What education is involved for someone to become a naturopath?

Currently, several ways exist in which someone may study to become a naturopath. Some naturopaths receive their degrees from accredited postgraduate colleges that are structured very much like medical schools. Other naturopathic programs are campus-based but not accredited. Nontraditional programs are available where people can learn the practice of naturopathic medicine through distance learning. Currently, no standardized training exists for naturopaths in the United States.

Q 19.7   How do I know that a naturopathic practitioner is reputable?

People can check with the Better Business Bureau to see whether any complaints have been logged about a particular naturopath in their area. It always is good for people to speak with someone who is familiar with the naturopath they are considering. People can call the office of a naturopath they are interested in visiting and ask about the practitioner's education and experience in treating health needs similar to theirs.

Q 19.8   I heard that naturopaths were illegal in my state. Is this true?

It depends on what the naturopath is doing. Being unlicensed is not the same as being illegal. In 2005, approximately one-fourth of the states in the United States offered licenses for naturopaths to practice naturopathic medicine (Cancer Cure Foundation, n.d.). It is not illegal for the naturopath to practice in a state where no license is offered, but the naturopath may not cross over into the practice of medicine, chiropractic, or acupuncture (unless already licensed under appropriate state boards). Once a state establishes licensure for naturopaths, then only naturopaths who are licensed by that particular state board of naturopathic medicine may practice and call themselves naturopathic doctors. In states that do not have licensure for naturopaths, naturopaths practice with restrictions in their scope and advertising. Without licensure, naturopaths do not have title protection to use the title "doctor" (in those states, they are called "naturopaths" or "naturopathic practitioners"). In states that do not offer licenses, it is legal to practice as a naturopath as long as the naturopath does not violate any existing laws or rules (a medical board law restricting the diagnosis and treatment of medical diseases to the practice of medicine).

19.9   Will my health insurance cover the cost of my visits to a naturopath?

Currently, health insurance probably will *not* cover the cost of visits to a naturopath or treatments recommended by the naturopath. Health insurance often is limited in regard to covering expenses for health promotion and generally does not cover the cost of nutritional supplements. Because of public demand, this situation may change as more and more people see the benefits of naturopathic care and realize they can improve their health using natural methods. More medical doctors are being educated in various aspects of naturopathic medicine and prefer to use the term "integrative medicine" to describe their practice. Some insurance companies may consider these doctors to be "out of network," but insurance may cover some portion of the visit. Individuals should check with their own health insurance provider for applicable coverage under their particular policy.

19.10   How can I afford naturopathic care if my health insurance doesn't cover it?

One strategy is for people to utilize a health or flexible savings account through their employer. The employer deducts a preset amount of money from the employee's wages; that money is used to reimburse the employee for his or her office visits, treatments, and supplements using pretax dollars. People should talk with the naturopathic provider they are considering to discuss costs and payment options.

19.11 Is a naturopath the same as a homeopath?

A naturopath also may be a homeopath, but a homeopath is not necessarily a naturopath. A homeopath usually practices only homeopathy. Some people think the term "homeopathy" is synonymous with the practice of natural medicine or herbal therapy, but that is not the case. Homeopathy is a very specific system of natural medicine developed approximately 200 years ago by German physician Samuel Hahnemann (Gerber, 2001). Hahnemann used highly diluted natural substances to stimulate the body to heal itself and had tremendous success with saving people from various epidemics and maladies in his day. Homeopaths today still practice homeopathy based on Hahnemann's basic principles and philosophy. A naturopath may choose to practice homeopathy in addition to many other modalities.

19.12 My chiropractor has recommended vitamins for me. How is a naturopath different from a chiropractor?

Important differences exist between the two professions. Naturopaths are educated in many natural therapeutic modalities, including methods of detoxification and nutritional counseling. Some chiropractors have an additional interest in nutrition or herbal therapy, but chiropractors' main focus is the spine, the musculoskeletal system, and the nervous system. Naturopaths are not legally permitted to do chiropractic spinal manipulations unless they have a license to practice chiropractic medicine.

19.13 I already have a "regular" doctor. How does naturopathic care fit in with what my doctor does now?

A medical doctor treats patients for a specific medical condition, whereas the naturopath's primary focus is increasing patients' overall health. Many patients who consult with naturopaths currently are seeing a medical doctor for one or more medical conditions. A naturopath does not replace a medical doctor. Naturopathic care involves looking for the underlying cause of patients' medical conditions or the reason their body became ill.

When using herbal therapy, naturopaths are aware of herb-drug interactions and can guide patients in the safe use of herbal therapy along with any prescribed medications they may be taking. Many medications deplete the body of important nutrients (for example, beta-blockers deplete coenzyme Q10, an important nutrient for heart health; and birth control pills and anticonvulsant medications deplete folic acid, an important nutrient to prevent many conditions, such as heart disease, Alzheimer disease, and cancer). Naturopaths take nutrient depletion from medications into consideration and will recommend supplements to maximize health and promote longevity.

Health conditions that are stress-related, such as acid reflux and hypertension, respond very well to a naturopathic approach using nutrition, herbal therapy, and dietary modifications. People who undergo surgical procedures and also participate in naturopathic care often recover more quickly with less reliance on postoperative pain medication.

Methods of Treatment

Q 19.14   What are the various natural methods that a naturopath uses?

Naturopaths are educated in a wide variety of natural methods, such as nutrition and vitamin therapy, herbal therapy, homeopathy, colonic irrigation and hydrotherapy (the use of water for healing), or reflexology (applying pressure to areas on hands, feet, or ears that correspond to internal organs). In addition, electrodermal screening (using computers to test skin response), hypnosis and visualization, traditional Chinese medicine and acupuncture, light and color therapy, Ayurvedic medicine (traditional medicine of India), ultrasonic and electrostimulation therapy, and flower essences and aromatherapy are some of the many different methods of natural healing that naturopaths might use.

Q 19.15   I'd like to stop taking some of my prescription medications. Can a naturopathic doctor help me to do that?

In some cases, naturopaths can help to improve patients' health to the extent that prescription medication may no longer be necessary, but naturopaths cannot advise patients to stop taking their medication. That is the responsibility of the prescribing physician. Serious consequences can result from stopping medication abruptly, so patients must discuss these matters with their medical doctor.

Q 19.16   I've seen an advertisement for a naturopath who does colon therapy. What is that?

Colon therapy, also known as colonics, is irrigation of the bowel using temperature-controlled filtered water. The irrigation is limited to the large intestine. The purpose is to promote healing through detoxification of the large intestine by removal of old fecal material.

Q 19.17   If I decide to try naturopathic care, will the naturopath want me to become a vegetarian?

This depends on the individual and the naturopath. Some naturopaths believe that health can only be achieved by avoiding all animal products, but this is not the case with all naturopaths. Although some people can be healthy on a vegetarian diet, others fare better when they include animal-based protein in their diet. All naturopaths agree on the benefits of organically grown foods. Many people have health problems related to milk products. Naturopathic practitioners may encourage patients to eliminate milk products to see whether their health improves. In any case, they often recommend increased consumption of fresh fruits and vegetables to promote health and longevity.

Q 19.18   I think many of my health issues are stress related. How can a naturopath help me with stress?

Stress may be present in a variety of ways. Most people think of stress as being related to feeling pressured or worried. Even people who may feel they have no stress can have an internal stress of which they have no conscious awareness. Anyone who has chronic pain, insomnia, allergies, or low blood sugar also experiences stress.

The standard American diet creates a great deal of internal stress because of problems related to poor blood-sugar control. Chronic low blood sugar causes the adrenal glands to become exhausted as a result of continual release of adrenaline and cortisol in an attempt to raise blood-sugar levels. A person with adrenal exhaustion is fatigued easily, craves sugar and salt, and is prone to respiratory infections and pneumonia. Unfortunately, as people become increasingly fatigued, they tend to reach for more sweets, caffeinated drinks, and fast foods that only make the condition worse. Naturopaths can help by suggesting dietary adjustments to maintain a healthy blood sugar level. Such adjustments include the elimination of caffeine, sugar, processed foods, hydrogenated oils (e.g., margarine), and products made from refined white flour.

Even if patients do not have a blood-sugar imbalance, naturopaths may help them to handle stress by suggesting the use of *adaptogens.* An adaptogen is an herb that has been shown to help the body to resist the damaging effects of stress—in other words, to adapt to stress. Some examples of adaptogenic herbs are *Ashwaganda, Schisandra,* and *Rhodiola rosea.* Each herb has a different way of helping a person to resist stress. Some adaptogens are more energizing, whereas others are more calming. Naturopaths find the adaptogenic herb that is right for the patient.

19.19   How would a naturopath know if I need an adaptogen?

A naturopath uses a hair analysis of tissue minerals to evaluate the body's ability to cope with stress. By comparing the ratios of various minerals in a patient's hair, the naturopath can find out if the person is in the early (alarm reaction) or late (burn out) stages of stress. Hair analysis often uncovers hidden stress issues of which patients may not be aware. Many naturopaths use hair analysis to evaluate stress as well as other conditions that can be helped through the use of proper diet and nutritional supplements.

19.20   I read a book written by a naturopath recommending different diets for different blood types. Does this approach really work?

The book being referred to is *Eat Right 4 Your Type* by naturopath James D'Adamo, ND (1997). D'Adamo recommended that people with blood type O eat animal protein and avoid wheat in all forms. D'Adamo believes people with blood type A do best on a vegetarian diet or vegetarian with fish diet. People with blood type B are supposed to tolerate dairy products very well but do not do well with chicken, among other foods. The diet for blood type AB seems to be the most restrictive diet to manage; the only meats D'Adamo recommended for this blood type were lamb and turkey. D'Adamo does not recommend pork for any of the blood types.

D'Adamo's (1997) blood type diets may work better for some people than others. In particular, people with blood type O often fare much better when they do not attempt to be vegetarian. Otherwise, individual results from the blood type diets are variable, and further research is needed to confirm D'Adamo's assertions.

Q 19.21   I am interested in losing weight. Can a naturopath help me to do this?

Improving health with weight management is one of the most common reasons people seek naturopathic care. Many people lose weight after consulting with a naturopath.

Often, overweight people struggle with sugar cravings because of poor digestion. It is very difficult to resist the quick energy that sugar provides when a person is unable to digest proteins and fats. A naturopath can assess whether a patient's digestion is adequate, based on his or her symptoms and other testing. Staying on a healthy eating plan is much easier when one has good digestion.

A common situation that some overweight women face is low thyroid function caused by an imbalance of female hormones, or *estrogen dominance*. They may even have normal thyroid hormone blood tests but still not have normal thyroid *function*. Unless the female hormonal imbalance is corrected, even thyroid replacement therapy is ineffective for weight management. This is a complex issue that requires specialized testing to treat. In many cases, people lose weight, increase their energy, and improve their health with naturopathic care.

References

Cancer Cure Foundation. (n.d.). *About naturopaths.* Retrieved September 2, 2005, from http://www.cancure.org/naturopaths.htm

D'Adamo, P. (with Whitney, C.). (1997). *Eat right 4 your type: The individualized diet solution to staying healthy, living longer and achieving your ideal weight.* New York: G.P. Putnam's Sons.

Gerber, R. (2001). *Vibrational medicine: The #1 handbook of subtle-energy therapies* (3rd ed.). Rochester, VT: Bear and Co.

Wood, M. (2000). *Vitalism: The history of herbalism, homeopathy, and flower essences* (2nd ed.). Berkeley, CA: North Atlantic Books.

Resources

American Association of Naturopathic Physicians: www.naturopathic.org

National Center for Complementary and Alternative Medicine, National Institutes of Health: http://nccam.nih.gov/health/homeopathy/

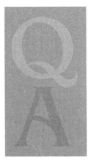

Chapter 20
Health Screening and Monitoring

Janis A. Cruce, MSN, RN, CS, FNP

Breast Health

Q 20.1 Why should I do breast self-exams (BSEs)? My breasts are so lumpy. I feel all kinds of lumps, and it scares me.

BSEs are very important in early detection of breast problems. Even though a woman's breasts are lumpy, any changes in her breasts can be detected. BSEs will get women to become familiar with their usual lumps and help them to detect changes. Women should ask their healthcare provider for assistance in how to best perform BSE.

Q 20.2 How often do women need to have screening mammograms done?

Major authorities vary on this recommendation. Many recommend starting at age 40, screening every one to two years thereafter until age 50, and then annually (Grosskreutz & Henshaw, 1999). Women should consult with their healthcare provider regarding the best recommendation for them.

Q 20.3 How often are mammograms recommended for women with breast implants?

Mammograms are recommended for women with breast implants on the same schedule as women without breast implants.

Q 20.4 I heard that mammograms can cause implants to rupture. Is that a reason not to have a mammogram done?

Little evidence supports that mammograms can cause breast implants to rupture, but there have been reported cases. Breast implants are not a contraindication for mammography. Women should continue to have mammograms done as part of breast cancer screening, along with regular BSE and clinical breast exams.

Q 20.5   When should mammograms be done on women who have a positive family history of breast cancer?

High-risk women who have a positive family history of breast cancer may start mammography at age 35, especially if breast cancer has been diagnosed before menopause in first-degree relatives.

Q 20.6   When should women have an ultrasound of the breast?

Ultrasounds of the breast are ordered for younger women, usually younger than age 30, or for women who are lactating or pregnant. Ultrasounds of the breast are considered as part of an evaluation of a mass or ambiguous mammogram report. Ultrasound is not a screening test that is done routinely. Ultrasounds can detect breast cysts and certain breast cancers.

Q 20.7   For those with fibrocystic breast disease, should mammograms be done earlier?

Fibrocystic breast disease does not require earlier screening with mammograms. It is very important, though, to get in the habit of doing regular BSEs as well as having a clinician do breast exams on a regular basis. It often is difficult to examine breast tissue that is fibrocystic, and knowing what "normal" feels like will help women to determine when something other than this is palpated.

Q 20.8   What does "BIRADS" mean?

"BIRADS" stands for the American College of Radiology Breast Imaging Reporting and Data System. The use of this system is mandatory to report results of mammograms. The categories range from 0–5. This allows a uniform reporting method so that different radiology reports can be compared.

Gynecologic Health

Q 20.9   How often do women need to have Pap smears done?

Women need to have Pap smears when they become sexually active or starting by age 21. After age 30, women who have had three negative Pap smears may be screened every two to three years (Yee, Baillie, Ho, Schapira, & Van Egeren, 2001). If women have any risk factors, such as being HIV positive or having a history of sexually transmitted diseases, they may need a Pap smear more often. Specific recommendations of major authorities vary, so women should talk to their healthcare provider regarding the best schedule for them.

20.10   Can a Pap smear detect whether I have ovarian cancer?

A Pap smear cannot detect ovarian cancer. Ovarian cancer and breast cancer in first-degree relatives may indicate a hereditary risk. Assessment for ovarian cancer requires evaluation by a healthcare provider.

20.11   What is a ThinPrep® (Cytyc, Marlborough, MA) Pap smear?

ThinPrep is a newer technology using a liquid solution for the cervical cells. It provides a better slide to view the cells and allows for further testing of abnormal cells. However, not enough evidence exists at this point to say it is a replacement for the traditional method of capturing cervical cells.

20.12   Does an abnormal Pap smear mean I have cancer?

An abnormal Pap smear does not mean a woman has cancer. Abnormal Pap smears need to be followed closely. The most common cause of abnormal Pap smears is the human papillomavirus (HPV). Certain strains of this virus can lead to cervical cancer. Close follow-up with repeat Pap smears can detect changes in cervical cells. Because many different treatment options are available, early detection is key to optimal reproductive health.

20.13   What does a colposcopy involve? Why do I need one?

Colposcopy involves the use of a machine that magnifies the cervix. It enables healthcare providers to assess lesions that are not visible with the naked eye.

20.14   Does a cervical biopsy hurt?

Cervical biopsy can cause a sudden cramping sensation. Some providers use a numbing medication, which also can sting. Other providers will do the biopsy without the numbing medication because the biopsy is so fast that the discomfort is thought to be about the same as that of the numbing medication. Women always should ask their provider if they have questions.

Q 20.15   Why do I need to have an endometrial biopsy done just because I am having vaginal bleeding?

Abnormal vaginal bleeding can be a sign of a serious problem. The endometrial biopsy can detect abnormal cells in the lining of the uterus.

Q 20.16   I am afraid of getting ovarian cancer. How can I be sure I do not have it?

Ovarian cancer only can be diagnosed by biopsy, but pelvic ultrasound can tell whether a problem exists. Pelvic ultrasound is not recommended to be done on a regular basis as a screening procedure. Women need to consult with their healthcare provider, especially if they have vague abdominal symptoms. A regular pelvic exam is a good place to start.

Q 20.17   Will uterine fibroids turn into cancer?

Uterine fibroids are usually benign. However, women with uterine fibroids are monitored for any rapid growth of fibroids or changes that may require further evaluation.

Treatments and Interventions

Q 20.18   What is a hysterectomy?

A hysterectomy is the surgical removal of the uterus. This is done through the abdomen or the vagina. A hysterectomy may or may not include removal of one or both ovaries.

Q 20.19   Once I've had a hysterectomy, will I have to take hormones?

If a woman has a hysterectomy and her ovaries are removed, hormones may be used in some cases to help to control immediate menopause symptoms. If one or both ovaries remain, then the woman will not go into surgical menopause; only her periods will stop. Women and their healthcare providers should discuss the benefits and risks of hormone replacement therapy related to their specific situation.

Q 20.20 **Why should I go to the doctor for a checkup? I've had a hysterectomy.**

Even if a woman has had a hysterectomy, she may need a pelvic exam. She will need a clinical breast exam, too. Many changes occur in women's general health as they mature, and they should discuss issues related to their health with their provider (U.S. Department of Health and Human Services Office of Public Health and Science, Office of Disease Prevention and Health Promotion, 1998). Women also will need to be evaluated for osteoporosis. Regular health monitoring is valuable for women of all ages.

Q 20.21 **When should I get a bone density test? Why should I get one?**

Sources recommend different ages for women to start screening for osteoporosis with a dual energy x-ray absorptiometry bone density test. The recommended age to start screening varies from 55–65. Bone scans are used to screen for risks for osteoporosis or loss of bone density and are painless. Women who have risk factors for osteoporosis should get a bone scan at a younger age.

Q 20.22 **Do I need to take extra calcium?**

A calcium intake of 1,200 mg per day, with vitamin D, is recommended for women older than age 50 (National Institutes of Health Office of Dietary Supplements, 2005). Women should assess their dietary intake of calcium to determine whether additional calcium intake is a good plan.

References

Grosskreutz, S., & Henshaw, D.C. (1999). Radiology. In B.J. Cayetano, B.S. Anderson, V.M. Pressler, L.J. Armstrong, C.K. Hughes, C.E. Minami, et al. (Eds.), *Diagnostic standards for early breast cancer: Primary care practitioner version* (pp. 1–4). Honolulu, HI: Hawaii Department of Health Breast and Cervical Cancer Control Program.

National Institutes of Health Office of Dietary Supplements. (2005). *Dietary supplement fact sheet: Calcium.* Retrieved August 1, 2005, from http://dietary-supplements.info.nih .gov/factsheets/calcium.asp

U.S. Department of Health and Human Services Office of Public Health and Science, Office of Disease Prevention and Health Promotion. (1998). *Clinician's handbook of preventive services: Put prevention into practice* (2nd ed.). Washington, DC: Author.

Yee, E.F., Baillie, S., Ho, M., Schapira, M., & Van Egeren, L. (Eds.). (2001). *Women's primary care guide.* Washington, DC: VHA Employee Education System.

Resource

Association of Women's Health, Obstetric and Neonatal Nurses: www.awhonn.org

Chapter 21

Nurses' Health Study Update

Graham A. Colditz, MD, DrPH

Background/Significance

21.1 What is the Nurses' Health Study?

The Nurses' Health Study is an ongoing cohort study. Investigators at Harvard University have been following 121,700 women since they volunteered to participate in the study in 1976 (Hankinson, Colditz, Manson, & Speizer, 2001). Women are followed with a questionnaire every two years. The questionnaire allows participants to update their information on lifestyle factors such as weight, diet, physical activity, smoking, and so forth, as well as the diagnosis of major illnesses. This resource allows the investigators to evaluate lifestyle in relation to a broad array of health conditions affecting middle-aged and older women.

21.2 What is the difference between the Nurses' Health Study and the Nurses' Health Study II?

Researchers began the Nurses' Health Study II in 1989 to address the relation between specific formulations of oral contraceptives and the risk of breast cancer. This younger generation of women had the opportunity to use oral contraceptives in adolescence and hence was able to use oral contraceptives for a far longer time than the women in the original Nurses' Health Study.

21.3 What time frame do the studies cover?

Women in the original Nurses' Health Study were born from 1922–1945 and in the Nurses' Health Study II, from 1946–1964. The study has allowed investigators to gather retrospective data dating to 1922. It also allows prospective data collection by following the same cohort of study participants as they age.

Q 21.4   How were people selected for the studies?

For both studies, the participants selected were RNs. The main purpose of this selection was to increase the efficiency of the study. The cost of conducting the study was kept at a minimum because women educated as RNs could more accurately report their medical conditions. A major expense of this study was confirming the illnesses among study participants. Fewer errors in reporting lead to an increase in accuracy and a reduction in cost.

Q 21.5   Are new people being added, or do the studies just follow current participants?

At this time, neither of these studies is adding new people. Researchers are following the same participants over time and continually updating the information they have on these participants.

Q 21.6   What is the goal of the studies?

The overall goal of the studies is to relate lifestyle factors to the development of chronic conditions. This will help researchers to identify strategies that help women reduce risks and maintain healthy lives.

Q 21.7   How do findings of the study compare with other studies, such as the Women's Health Initiative?

In general, the results from the Nurses' Health Study compare favorably with other major investigations. For example, researchers in the Nurses' Health Study see the same relationship among overweight, obesity, and cancer risk as that reported by the American Cancer Society's Cancer Prevention Study II. With regard to hormones, a reduced risk of colon cancer, a reduced risk of fractures, and an increased risk of breast cancer are seen in this study as in the Women's Health Initiative. With regard to heart disease, researchers have seen a reduced risk with use of postmenopausal hormones that has not been observed in the Women's Health Initiative, which used one single formulation, a combined estrogen plus progestin pill.

Q 21.8   How are the studies funded?

Throughout the Nurses' Health Study and the Nurses' Health Study II, funding has been primarily through the National Cancer Institute. Other institutes at the National Institutes of Health provide additional funding to study specific conditions such as diabetes, heart disease, and fractures.

 21.9   Can a participant leave the studies at any time?

From time to time, participants indicate that they are too busy to complete a questionnaire. Many request to be included in subsequent years. However, on rare occasions, participants have asked to be removed from the studies, and the researchers honor this request.

 21.10   How is confidentiality of questionnaire data maintained?

The use of identification numbers and the storage of data by this coded number maintain the confidentiality of questionnaire data. Data on exposure and outcomes are maintained in a secure system and only are linked to the name and address file when researchers need to contact the participants, either to mail a questionnaire or to confirm a reported major illness.

 21.11   How are findings of the studies shared with the public?

Findings from the studies are shared with the public in a number of ways. Local media often cover major medical journal articles. Researchers have prepared a book summarizing the major findings that has had wide circulation (Hankinson et al., 2001). The investigators also travel to scientific meetings and to gatherings of RNs to present updates on the study. All participants in this study receive an annual newsletter in which the investigators highlight major recent findings.

 21.12   I get your newsletter. Can I use information published in it for the patient education I provide, or do I need copyright permission?

Information in the newsletter is freely available for use by participants in the study if they find that it could be useful in their work.

Future Implications

 21.13   Is there an end date planned, or will the study continue into the future?

The study is ongoing and is dependent on funding from the National Cancer Institute. This funding is primarily contingent on having scientific investigation of sufficient quality to justify the expense. At this stage, no planned end date exists.

Q 21.14   Have the study findings brought about any changes in health policy or recommendations for patient care based on study findings?

Findings from the study clearly have had an impact on prevention recommendations that are widely disseminated. The study's findings on alcohol and breast cancer have affected recommendations for women, and findings on physical activity and prevention of heart disease, diabetes, and breast cancer support national recommendations. Other findings in relation to diet and the health effects of postmenopausal hormones clearly feed into the counseling that primary care providers share with their patients when considering risks and benefits.

Reference

Hankinson, S.E., Colditz, G.A., Manson, J.E., & Speizer, F.E. (Eds.). (2001). *Healthy women, healthy lives: A guide to preventing disease, from the landmark Nurses' Health Study.* New York: Simon & Schuster.

Resource

Nurses' Health Study Web site: www.channing.harvard.edu/nhs

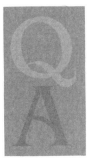

Chapter 22
Stress Management

Jacqueline M. Loversidge, MS, RN, C

Background

 22.1 What is stress?

"Stress" is a term used to describe the body's reaction to a circumstance that an individual perceives as a threat. The threat can be emotional, such as the feeling one might have while engaged in an argument, or it can be physical, such as the feeling one might get when involved in a near-accident in a car, or even the physical stress felt during a bad cold or flu. Stress is different for everyone, so the word "perception" is key.

Stress can be "good," for example, the heightened arousal one might feel before a wedding, birth, start of a new job, giving a presentation, or graduation. "Distress" is negative stress and covers the gamut of the physical, emotional or mental, and spiritual arenas. Most people, over the period of their lives, have developed skills to cope with short-term stressors. It is chronic distress that has long-term negative effects on the mind and body (Benson & Stuart, 1992).

22.2 What is the mind/body connection, and how is it related to stress?

The term "mind/body connection" implies that the mind and body are one and that they are related to circumstances in a person's life and environment. So, for example, if someone were at risk for heart disease, that person could positively alter his or her risk by engaging in healthy behaviors known to have an effect on heart health, such as nutrition, exercise, and stress management. Inherent in the notion of interconnectedness between mind and body is a sense of control or power over the biology of belief (Benson, 1997), which can give a person a sense of authority about one's ability to have an impact on his or her overall health.

A growing body of scientific research exists in this area, called psychoneuroimmunology. The more scientists understand about the body's reaction to accumulated stress hormones, the better equipped healthcare providers will be to help people to manage chronic health problems that have some stress-related components.

Q 22.3   When I feel stressed, what is happening in my body?

The stress response occurs when the body automatically reacts to circumstances that are perceived as a physical or emotional threat. When this happens, the body responds as though the threat will affect the individual's life or safety. This is a primal response, during which a person's brain sends chemical signals to the body to release stress hormones so that he or she can react to the threat. The stress hormones put the individual on alert, resulting in more focused concentration, faster reaction time, increased blood pressure, and increased strength and agility. What people immediately recognize are the pounding heart, speeded breathing, and sweaty palms. This is known as the "fight-or-flight" response (Benson & Stuart, 1992).

Q 22.4   What are the stress hormones, and what do they do?

Scientists still are unraveling the complex mechanisms that come into play during the stress response. The stress circuit, known as the hypothalamic-pituitary-adrenal axis, explains a number of stress-related conditions. In response to a stressor, the hypothalamus releases a stress hormone called corticotropin-releasing hormone (CRH). This hormone stimulates the pituitary gland to release an additional hormone, adrenocorticotropin (ACTH), into the bloodstream. ACTH stimulates the adrenal glands to release additional stress hormones (National Institutes of Health [NIH], 2002).

The stress hormones include epinephrine (adrenaline), norepinephrine (noradrenaline), and cortisol. All three of these hormones act together in response to a stressor. Epinephrine is the hormone responsible for increased heart rate and blood pressure and faster reaction time. Cortisol, a glucocorticoid, releases sugar as glucose. The glucose serves as fuel for the brain and the muscles. Under normal circumstances, cortisol shuts down the stress response when the threat has passed by influencing the hypothalamus to stop production of CRH. When an individual experiences chronic stress, this feedback effect fails to take place (NIH, 2002).

In response to stress, the brain also secretes endorphins, which are pain-killing hormones known as the body's "natural morphine." Also, the immune system responds in the event that it is needed to fight infection, and platelets in the blood become stickier, making clotting more efficient (Benson & Stuart, 1992).

This is a healthy, natural response designed to protect people from what their physiology interprets as danger. However, when people remain in a state of heightened arousal or chronic stress, a number of long-term effects begin to take place. The inside of the arteries can be damaged by the turbulent blood flow caused by high blood pressure, increasing the risk for heart disease as well as for other problems related to hypertension. Some of the body's ongoing functions are put on hold, such as digestion and reproduction, so that all of the body's energy can focus on dealing with the stress. Elevated cortisol levels also have been associated with increased abdominal fat, bone loss, damage to memory cells, and interruption of normal function of the immune system (Benson & Stuart, 1992; Davis, Eshelman, & McKay, 2000; Elkin, 1999).

Q 22.5   Does a relationship exist between stress and weight management?

A growing body of science is exploring this relationship. Excessive amounts of the stress hormone cortisol have been related to sleep disturbances and an increased risk for accumulation of abdominal fat. In addition, a relationship appears to exist between getting too little sleep (less than seven or eight hours per night of continuous sleep) and an increase in cortisol levels. Research on children and adolescents has demonstrated that too little sleep is related to obesity in children. The elevated cortisol levels associated with stress, including insufficient sleep, may have the effect of fooling people's bodies into thinking they are in famine. The body stores fat more efficiently as a protective mechanism. Abdominal fat and obesity, in particular, have been linked to a number of diseases, especially an increased risk for heart disease (NIH, 2002).

Q 22.6   Is there any relationship between stress and disease?

Scientists have been reluctant to state that a true cause and effect exists between stress and disease. However, research has shown that there are a number of associations between stress and certain diseases or conditions. Activation of the stress system, especially if it is long term, can increase the risk of atherosclerotic heart disease and other forms of cardiovascular disease, as well as depression. In addition, people with long periods of excessive amounts of cortisol secretion may experience suppression of thyroid hormones and suppression of the immune system. Because these individuals are at higher risk for these health problems, they are likely to have a shortened life span, by as much as 15–20 years, if they are not treated (NIH, 2002).

In addition to physical problems, stress plays an important role in performance and efficiency. As stress levels increase to a manageable degree, performance generally increases. Just ask those who work best with a deadline. However, if stress levels increase to the point that the person cannot cope, performance levels fall dramatically (Benson & Stuart, 1992; Davis et al., 2000; Elkin, 1999).

Q 22.7   What are the signs of stress? How will I know when I am not coping well?

Warning signs of stress can fall into a number of categories, including physical or emotional symptoms, problem behaviors, and distorted thinking. Examples include (Benson & Stuart, 1992; Davis et al., 2000; Elkin, 1999)

- Physical symptoms (headache, sweaty palms, fatigue, racing heart, quickened breath, tight neck and shoulders, indigestion, stomachaches, "butterflies" in the stomach)
- Behavioral symptoms (smoking, alcohol abuse, inability to accomplish tasks, difficulty with relationships)
- Emotional symptoms (crying, anger, depression, loneliness, feeling powerless, feeling bored or edgy)
- Cognitive symptoms (difficulty thinking clearly, feeling worried, loss of sense of humor, forgetfulness, inability to make decisions).

People will know they are not coping well if their stress symptoms continue. The physical signs people feel when experiencing an "in-the-moment" stressor and the signs they feel when they have been stressed continuously may be different. For example, a mother with a child who is a constant discipline challenge may find that she is continuously on edge. Signs of ineffective coping might include being sad or depressed, feeling angry all the time, becoming tearful easily, having insomnia, losing appetite, or feeling isolated from friends and family. Again, people all react a bit differently, so being aware of patterns of emotional or physical discomfort related to stress is extremely important. This is called "stress awareness" (Benson & Stuart, 1992).

Interventions

Q 22.8 **Are there any skills I can learn to quickly feel better in a stressful moment?**

People can learn a number of skills to help relieve the symptoms associated with the initiation of fight-or-flight symptoms. These are very quick and easy to use and can be done in almost any situation. In particular, two techniques exist that involve using the breath. One is abdominal breathing, or "belly breathing." The other is called a "mini," or mini relaxation response (Benson & Stuart, 1992).

Q 22.9 **What does "using the breath" mean? How is that done, and what does it accomplish?**

"Using the breath" refers to a method of relaxation that uses the breath as a mental focal point. If people are paying attention to their breathing, it will be easier to calm down, gain mental focus, and be better able to deal with whatever stressor they are facing. When people are tense, they tend to breathe shallowly and in the chest. Belly breathing, deep and into the abdomen, has been shown to effectively reduce anxiety, irritability, and muscle tension. Practice by sitting or lying comfortably. People can close their eyes if they are comfortable doing so. Individuals place their hands on their abdomen and focus their attention on their breathing. Notice how the abdomen rises with the inhalation and falls with the exhalation. When performing belly breathing, people should focus their mind on their breathing, tuning out intruding thoughts as best they can.

Minis, or mini relaxation exercises, use the technique involved in abdominal breathing. One example of a mini includes slowly counting from 10 down to zero, saying one number at a time to oneself on each exhale. Another way to do a mini is to repeat slowly to oneself, "one, two, three, four" on the in-breath and "four, three, two, one" on the out-breath. Instead of numbers, some may prefer to repeat a short prayer. For those who are not fond of airplane flights, these are wonderful methods to keep a sense of calm on takeoff and landing.

People may find that they prefer either abdominal breathing alone or combining an additional mental focus or mini. If people have a "busy mind," they may find that the addition of numbers or another focus will help them to tune out everyday thoughts and relax more effectively.

Q 22.10   Is meditation the same as "the relaxation response"?

Dr. Herbert Benson first identified the relaxation response as a counterbalancing mechanism to the fight-or-flight response. Meditation is one of the many techniques that elicit this response. The relaxation response is a state of profound, deep rest, different from sleep, that can be intentionally elicited by using any of a variety of techniques to neutralize the effects of stress hormones. The relaxation response must be elicited for a minimum of 10–20 minutes for the neutralization effect to take place. The relaxation response has the effect of decreasing the heart rate, decreasing the breathing rate, lowering the blood pressure, slowing the metabolism, and decreasing muscle tension.

Regular practice for 10–20 minutes once or twice daily seems to have positive effects on diseases or conditions that are related to or affected by stress. In addition, practitioners of the relaxation response report a decrease in stress-related symptoms, decreased anxiety, increased concentration and awareness, better sleep, freedom from negative thoughts, and enhanced performance and efficiency (Benson & Stuart, 1992).

Q 22.11   How can I elicit the relaxation response?

All of the techniques involve some kind of a mental focus, and all produce a reduction in heart rate, breathing rate, blood pressure, muscle tension, and metabolism. Examples of these techniques include

- Meditation—uses a word, phrase, short prayer, or mantra as the mental focus
- Visualization or guided imagery—uses the imagination and may involve all five senses. This might include imagining a beautiful, peaceful scene in detail (e.g., a meadow with soft grass under foot, a fresh breeze on the skin, a blue sky) or imagining a healing light flowing through the body.
- Abdominal breathing—uses the breath as the mental focus
- Mindfulness—the practice of being in the moment

- Progressive relaxation—the use of muscle tension and relaxation, sequencing progressively throughout the body, often from head to toe
- Yoga or Tai Chi—uses asanas (poses) and/or movement as the mental focus. The more active forms of yoga, such as ashtanga (power) yoga, will raise a person's vital signs during the more vigorous series of asanas, but the aftereffect is elicitation of the relaxation response.
- Aerobic (cardiovascular) exercise—Although heart rate, blood pressure, breathing rate, and metabolism all rise during exercise, similar to power yoga, the aftereffect can be similar to having elicited the relaxation response with more quieting methods.

Q 22.12   Explain "progressive relaxation."

Progressive relaxation, one of the methods of eliciting the relaxation response, relies on a person's ability to identify the difference between muscle tension and relaxation. It usually is done by first lying down in a comfortable position or by sitting comfortably in a chair with feet resting on the floor. Each muscle group is tensed for about five seconds and then intentionally relaxed. It is important to try to focus on one muscle group at a time. Practice by progressively tensing and relaxing the following muscle groups.

- Hands, forearms, and upper arms
- Head, face, throat, and shoulders, giving attention to the forehead, eyes, cheeks, jaw, and neck
- Chest, abdomen, and lower back
- Buttocks, thighs, calves, and feet

Q 22.13   How do I meditate?

Meditation is the practice of focusing one's attention on one thing at a time. Repeat, either out loud or silently, a word, syllable, sound (such as "ohm"), or phrase, such as a short prayer. If people choose to keep their eyes open during meditation, finding a visual focal point is also helpful. Follow this process:

- Find a comfortable position in a safe place. People may sit in a comfortable chair or lie down on the floor.
- Accept the fact that distracting thoughts will come into one's mind. When that happens, uncritically accept the fact that the thoughts are there, let them go, and come back to the focus.
- Meditate for a minimum of 10–20 minutes. People may meditate for a longer period of time, but this minimum, practiced once

or twice a day, likely will yield all the benefits of the relaxation response (Benson & Stuart, 1992; Carrington, 1998; Davis et al., 2000; Elkin, 1999).

22.14   **Describe "being mindful." How will accomplishing mindfulness help to relieve my stress?**

Mindfulness is the practice of "being in the moment." It is a letting go of the past and future and paying attention to what is in the here and now (Carrington, 1998; Kabat-Zinn, 1990, 1994; Nhat Hanh, 1987). In their everyday lives, people often are mentally ruminating about something distressing or unpleasant that already has occurred or worrying about and anticipating something that might happen. People spend much of their time being mentally somewhere other than where they are.

Most people can think of a time when they have been introduced to someone and then immediately forgot his or her name, or when they have completely lost their train of thought during a conversation. Most people have had the experience of reading a couple of paragraphs and having no recollection of the content. Reading comprehension ability is probably not at issue—more likely, their thoughts just traveled to another time and place. These moments exemplify *not* being mindful.

To practice mindfulness, one simply should be where he or she is. Here are several exercises for people to try.
- Pay close attention to someone they care about during a conversation.
- Take a walk, noticing everything around them and inside of them . . . the color of the sky, the temperature of the air, whether there is a breeze, or any sounds. Notice how their body feels; notice their breath moving in and out.
- Pay attention to a small child at play.
- Eat mindfully. Be mindful during a whole meal, paying attention to the flavors, textures, and smell of the food. Or they may be mindful with just one item, such as a piece of luscious chocolate. If people eat mindfully, they probably will eat more slowly and feel full more quickly—an added benefit!

22.15   **Are yoga and Tai Chi effective stress management tools? How do they help to relieve stress?**

Yoga and Tai Chi are meditative forms of exercise that Eastern cultures have practiced for centuries. The stress management benefits come from the fact that to practice the exercises properly, attention must be paid to the movements, forms, or poses (asanas) used in the practice. When people assume a yoga pose that requires balance and stretching, for example, it is difficult for their mind to move on to everyday distracting thoughts. Therefore, mindfulness is inherent in these practices.

22.16   What is imagery or visualization, and how is it done?

Imagery or visualization uses the imagination to elicit the relaxation response and to affect attitudes and behaviors. Imagery can be used to break out of negative thinking and replace those thoughts with positive images. All five senses can be evoked through the use of imagery (Benson & Stuart, 1992; Levine, 1991). Imagery is very personal, so people must practice with different images to see what is most effective for them. Some examples of imaging different sensations include the smell of the ocean; the smell of fresh-cut grass; the taste of garlic, chocolate, or lemon; the sound of birds singing; or the sight of a beautiful ocean, mountain, or forest scene.

Some individuals who practice imagery or visualization imagine a safe place and return mentally to that image during stressful times.

22.17   What is biofeedback, and how is it used to manage stress?

Biofeedback involves the use of technology—usually monitors—to measure physical changes brought about by the relaxation response. Monitors may measure heart rate, blood pressure, or skin temperature and give people a measurable account of how successful they are in their relaxation practice. Once people become accustomed to noticing how their body feels, they replace the use of monitors with astute body awareness.

Simple, inexpensive, and fun biofeedback monitors come in the form of "biodots," or stress cards that are made in the shape of credit cards. These gadgets use the same technology found in mood rings, which have gained renewed popularity. Mood rings, mood necklaces, and other jewelry can be found easily in inexpensive accessory stores in almost every mall. The chemical in these items changes colors in response to changes in body temperature. Biodots are worn on the hand, usually in the webbed area between the thumb and index finger. Stress cards are equipped with a small gel-pad that is pressed with the thumb. The science behind this simple technology is that when people are in a fight-or-flight mode, the blood vessels in their hands constrict, resulting in cold, clammy hands. As people relax, those blood vessels dilate, bringing more warm blood to the hands and increasing their temperature. Biodots simply help beginners become more aware of their body response and recognize that the physical changes brought about by the relaxation response are real and measurable.

Q 22.18   Sometimes I seem to "get myself into a tizzy," and the more I think about something stressful, the more stressed I become. The more stressed I become, the worse I feel. It is a vicious circle, and I cannot seem to get myself out of it. What can I do to improve the way I feel?

The "tizzy" described is called negative thinking. Negative thoughts often are automatic, knee-jerk responses to situations in which people feel out of control. A difficult realization is that most automatic negative thoughts are distorted, exaggerated, or illogical (Burns, 1990, 1993). All people want to believe that they are rational all of the time, but the fact is that when people are stressed, being rational can be very difficult. This is a prime example of the mind/body connection; when a person's *thinking* is negative, the fight-or-flight response kicks in.

Cognitive therapy is an approach to coping positively with negative thoughts. Burns (1990, 1993) has written workbooks anyone can use to master this technique. Cognitive therapy is built on the two major premises that much of people's stress comes from the way they think about or perceive a situation and that the thoughts that cause people stress usually are negative, unrealistic, and distorted.

The secret to feeling better when having automatic negative thinking is for people to *recognize* that their thoughts are distorted, then to challenge those thoughts. People should try to see their thoughts as though they were a compassionate, unbiased observer. Individuals should ask themselves if their thoughts really are true or if they are jumping to conclusions and also should ask themselves what is the worst that could happen. Look for key words in thinking, such as *should, must, always,* and *never.*

If people can identify their thoughts as distorted or irrational, they must reframe those thoughts so that they become more positive but truly real and believable. It does no good to try to "trick" oneself into a more positive way of thinking. People will find that as they reframe their thoughts, their stress symptoms will decrease, and their distress will lessen (Benson & Stuart, 1992; Burns, 1990, 1993; Davis et al., 2000; Elkin, 1999).

22.19   Is there any science behind the notion that writing things down can help to relieve feelings of stress? Are there any guidelines to doing this in an effective way?

Writing down one's innermost thoughts, known as "journaling," can improve an individual's health and feelings of well-being. Dr. James Pennebaker (1991) found that people who kept meaningful journals found their moods improved. The same people also sought health care for physical symptoms less often and had improved immune function. The same results did not occur if the person only kept notes on superficial subjects.

People should try journaling using these guidelines, gleaned from Pennebaker's (1991) work.
- Write for at least 15 minutes.
- Write about anything in their life that they are dwelling on or that is causing distress.
- Write about both the objective experience *and* their feelings.
- Do not worry about grammar or spelling.
- Write only to oneself, not with the intention of showing the journal to anyone else.
- If feeling overly distraught, stop and try a more gradual approach to the topic.
- Be aware that sad or depressed feelings may emerge immediately afterward. These feelings usually go away within an hour and rarely last longer than two days. Usually people feel relieved, content, and happy up to six months afterward.

22.20   Even during stressful times, if something strikes me as funny and I have a good laugh, I feel better. Is this healthy and appropriate?

Absolutely! Humor can be a wonderful stress management tool. Humor gives people a break from stress, restores emotional resources, and helps to sustain them so that they are better able to cope. Humor has been shown to enhance immune function and productivity. People who use humor as a positive coping strategy often are optimists, and optimism has been associated with longevity and better health (Benson & Stuart, 1992).

Q22.21   How important are close relationships with others when it comes to managing stress?

Close relationships with others can be a great source of comfort. Family, friends, and coworkers all can be a part of one's social network and can be of help during times of stress. It can be very helpful to talk things out with a trusted companion who is a good listener, offers objective perspectives, and is, in a word, therapeutic. Research has shown that people with strong social ties are healthier and live longer (Ornish, 1998).

Many people report that much of their stress comes from difficult relationships and poor communication. Working on assertive communication skills and letting people close to them know what they need in a relationship are important tools to help individuals in managing their stress.

Q22.22   Can time management strategies help a person to feel less stressed?

Yes, time management can help people to gain a better sense of control and help them focus on the things that are most important. Women especially try to "do it all," managing their own time as well as their family's activities and needs. Finding balance can be difficult.

People should identify where their time is spent. Are they spending time performing tasks that are unimportant? Are the items at the top of their "to-do" list truly important? Is their importance a reality, an illusion, or a designation assigned by someone else? *People's time should be spent on activities that are important to them.* If the tasks are not important, let them go. Individuals may need to be assertive with others who would fill up their day. Learning how to say "no" to peforming the task, while honoring the person who has asked, is a skill that takes some practice but will go a long way toward helping people manage their time and stress level.

Another strategy in managing time is for people to determine whether they can influence the object of their concern. Worrying about something one cannot change is counterproductive. Instead, people need to focus on what they can change or otherwise influence and set aside time to plan how they will go about accomplishing that objective (Covey, Merrill, & Merrill, 1995).

Q 22.23   If stress management techniques fail to be effective, and feelings of being overly stressed, sad, or angry remain, what is the next step?

If people have tried all the skills in their arsenal, have talked about the source of their stress with a trusted companion, and still are feeling distressed or sad, it may be wise to seek professional help. It is unwise to assume that feelings may resolve without intervention. It may be judicious to seek the care and counsel of their healthcare provider or a mental health professional.

Q 22.24   Can I expect to ever be stress free?

No one will ever be stress free. Stress is a natural part of life. The secret is in learning and practicing effective coping strategies so that people are prepared to meet the challenges of life head on. Also, by learning to engage effective coping mechanisms, individuals will enable themselves to harness their energies to gain a higher level of productivity and personal well-being (Benson & Proctor, 2003).

Q 22.25   What suggestions might be helpful when I have virtually no time to take care of myself?

People can reflect on what is important in their life. Is it their family, health, work, money, social network, or perhaps political affiliations? Many women believe it is their role and responsibility to be all things, to all people, all of the time. Although they know this simply is not possible, they often feel compelled to attempt to achieve an unrealistic and unreasonable ideal.

People must make sure their basic health needs are met. Are they getting enough sleep? Are they eating healthy foods? Are they getting enough nonsleep rest, relaxation, and physical exercise? Are their emotional needs being met? If the answer to any of these questions is no, consider what it would take to establish a plan that would better meet those needs. This may involve scheduling time for themselves and asking for support from their friends and family to help them to get what they need.

Q 22.26   What strategies can keep me feeling good about myself and my stress reactions managed?

One should think of a stress management plan as he or she would any healthy behavior. To stay on track, people need to make it a priority and have a plan. People who have ever tried to exercise, lose weight, or stop smoking may remember that they might have done really well as they got started, but then might have gotten stuck or had gone back to old habits when their guard was down.

Perhaps an individual has begun a daily relaxation response practice. All goes well for the first two months, then one day her family's needs interfere with her schedule, and she does not practice for two days. The individual may be at risk for a "lapse" or a "relapse." The science underpinning relapse prevention is grounded in cognitive-behavioral models (Larimer, Palmer, & Marlatt, 1999).

A lapse is a *temporary* deviation from the original plan. Everyone has lapses from time to time. It is important to see them as single events, learn from them, and move on. People must not allow a lapse to put them into a negative emotional state—see it as a learning opportunity, put it behind oneself, and move on.

A relapse, however, is a *pattern* of returning to the unhealthy habit. The majority of relapses come from four sources:
- Negative emotional states, including anger, anxiety, depression, frustration, and boredom: These are associated with the highest rate of relapse.
- Situations involving another person or a group of people: They often involve interpersonal conflict and may serve as triggers for more than half of all relapse episodes.
- Social pressure: This may include both direct verbal or nonverbal persuasion and indirect pressure (for example, being around other people who are engaged in the behavior to be avoided, such as smoking or drinking alcoholic beverages). These states have accounted for more than 20% of relapse episodes.
- Positive emotional states, such as celebrations: These states provide for exposure to cues to engage in celebratory behavior, such as alcohol consumption or other cravings.

To prevent a relapse, people need to plan for those times that they are most likely to feel stressed and stray from their plan. A deadline at work, family events, holidays, and even vacations can raise one's stress level. Anticipate and make a list of several personal high-risk situations, and include details such as names and places. Then make decisions about what to do to cope during those times. Decide what stress management skills to use under what circumstances and when to use them. Providing as much detail in the plan as possible will enable individuals to be in the best position to remain stress hardy.

References

Benson, H. (1997). *Timeless healing: The power and biology of belief.* New York: Simon & Schuster.

Benson, H., & Proctor, W. (2003). *The break-out principle: How to activate the natural trigger that maximizes creativity, athletic performance, productivity and personal well-being.* New York: Simon & Schuster.

Benson, H., & Stuart, E. (1992). *The wellness book: The comprehensive guide to maintaining health and treating stress-related illness.* New York: Simon & Schuster.

Burns, D.D. (1990). *The feeling good handbook.* New York: Plume.

Burns, D.D. (1993). *Ten days to self-esteem.* New York: Quill.

Carrington, P. (1998). *The book of meditation: The complete guide to modern meditation.* Boston: Element.

Covey, S.R., Merrill, A.R., & Merrill, R.A. (1995). *First things first: To live, to love, to learn, to leave a legacy.* New York: Simon & Schuster.

Davis, M., Eshelman, E.R., & McKay, M. (2000). *The relaxation and stress reduction workbook* (5th ed.). Oakland, CA: New Harbinger Publications.

Elkin, A. (1999). *Stress management for dummies.* Foster City, CA: IDG Books Worldwide.

Kabat-Zinn, J. (1990). *Full catastrophe living: Using the wisdom of your body and mind to face stress, pain, and illness.* New York: Bantam Doubleday Dell Publishing Group.

Kabat-Zinn, J. (1994). *Wherever you go, there you are: Mindfulness meditation in everyday life.* New York: Hyperion.

Larimer, M.E., Palmer, R.S., & Marlatt, G.A. (1999). Relapse prevention: An overview of Marlatt's cognitive-behavioral model. *Alcohol Research and Health, 23,* 151–160.

Levine, S. (1991). *Guided meditations, explorations and healings.* New York: Doubleday.

National Institutes of Health. (2002, September). *Stress system malfunction could lead to serious, life threatening disease.* Retrieved July 27, 2005, from http://www.nih.gov/news/pr/sep2002/nichd-09.htm

Nhat Hanh, T. (1987). *Being peace.* Berkeley, CA: Parallax Press.

Ornish, D. (1998). *Love and survival: The scientific basis for the healing power of intimacy.* New York: HarperCollins.

Pennebaker, J.W. (1991). Writing your wrongs. *American Health, 10,* 64–67.

Resources

National Institutes of Health: www.nih.gov
National Institute of Mental Health, National Institutes of Health: www.nimh.nih.gov

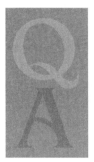

Chapter 23
Using Time Effectively

LeaRae Galarowicz, MS, RN, BC

Patient Care Challenges

Q 23.1 **What is the secret for organizing my clinical work so that I have enough time to get everything done for my patients?**

Planning is very important, both before starting work and then replanning whenever a significant change occurs in the day's events, such as a new admission or a patient crisis. A worksheet that lists patients' names, diagnoses, treatments, etc., and that has ample space for note-taking can be a valuable tool to help nurses to organize. Actively use the worksheet by highlighting priorities with a colored pen, crossing off completed tasks, and recording assessment data, symptoms, and lab results (Eckman & Newman, 1997). Keep the worksheet as a ready reference for questions from coworkers and family members as well as for documentation purposes. Do not forget to arrive at work in plenty of time to plan and prepare—it will be worth it in the long run.

Q 23.2 **Can you offer any helpful suggestions for organizing patient information that I gather during my shift so that it is easier to chart and update physicians and family members about a patient's condition?**

Many nurses find that carrying a worksheet during their shift not only serves as a reference for medication and treatment times but also, if actively used, can be a resource for lab and other test results, vital signs measurements, and assessment data. Organize the worksheet so that there is ample room for listing procedures and care information as well as for recording all significant data about each patient. Because the worksheet contains a great deal of important and confidential information, always know where it is and keep it secured from those who are not authorized to see it. Then, when nurses are asked for information about one of their patients or when it is time to chart, the worksheet will be an easily available and handy resource.

23.3 When we are short staffed and super busy, how do I determine what is most important to do for each of my patients?

Limited time and resources means that nurses will need to aim for what *really* matters. Focus on the essential and most important care/treatments for each patient. The newly admitted and those with unstable conditions will require closer observation. When setting priorities, nurses should ask themselves: What nursing measures will make the greatest difference in helping my patients to recover or heal? The answer may be to administer the antibiotic at the scheduled time, to monitor the circulation in the extremity, or to check the glucose level, depending upon the patient's diagnosis and status.

23.4 All day long I try to work as fast and efficiently as I can, but I never seem to be able to leave work on time. I am getting burned out! Any suggestions?

Busy workdays demand that nurses all work smarter, not harder. As nurses begin their workday by gathering information about all that needs to be done for their patients, they should plan ahead and cluster their activities to conserve their energy and that of their patients. One must remember to delegate routine, low-priority tasks in order to focus on measures that are more important. Nurses can ask others to help be their "eyes and ears" by checking on their patients when they are nearby and then reporting back to the nurse. Then, at the end of each day, nurses should take a few minutes to critique their day, evaluating how they might have streamlined their responsibilities more effectively. This will provide a jumpstart for tomorrow.

23.5 Do you have any hints to make it easier for me to ask others for help with managing patient care?

Delegating appropriately sends a message to nurses' coworkers and nursing assistants that they trust their skills, and it frees them to deal with activities of higher priority. It is both unnecessary and unwise for nurses to try to do everything themselves. They will not only be very busy, but they are likely to become overwhelmed and frustrated. Keep in mind the principles of effective and safe delegation: Delegate only to someone who is authorized and trained to do the task; carefully communicate instructions as to what needs to be done and

when to do it; and follow up by asking the recipient of the delegation to report how the patient tolerated the procedure as well as the
specific outcomes or results (Cook, Strauss, & Noelke, 2004).

Career Challenges

Q 23.6 **I have a tendency to overschedule myself by volunteering for special
projects and later worrying how I will be able to do everything I said
I would do. How can I learn to say no?**

Instead of responding immediately with a yes or no, make it a
rule to always "buy time" before agreeing to a new commitment.
Stepping aside affords nurses the opportunity to take a realistic
look at their current responsibilities as well as to consider important future events that will require their time and energy. Asking
for time before making a decision also allows them to determine
whether the request fits in with their priorities. When saying no,
one approach is for nurses to begin by explaining to others that
they believe their cause to be very worthy and that they certainly
would enjoy being involved, but that they are unable to help. Always try to avoid offering a specific reason for refusing—for example, having no personal e-mail account. The person requesting
help may refute the reason, such as offering to set up an e-mail
account for the individual, thereby making it even more difficult
for the individual to stand firm with her "no" answer (Cook et
al., 2004).

Q 23.7 **I've just accepted a new position as case manager and will be working
out of my home. Any tips to help me to be productive when I'll be
surrounded by so many distractions?**

Hawke (2002) offered these suggestions for telecommuting. Working out of one's home requires two important characteristics: self-
motivation and discipline. Begin by segregating some work space
from the home space. Next, individuals should organize the workspace so that they have all of their supplies at hand and ready for
use. The employee should prepare her family by alerting them to
the fact that when she is at her desk working, she is unavailable for
routine household chores and should be interrupted only if there is
an emergency. Resist the impulse to work in pajamas or loungewear,
as this may be sending oneself a subliminal message that this is relaxation time rather than work time. This can impede productivity.

Last, refuse to do any housework, such as emptying the dishwasher or doing a load of laundry, during one's scheduled work time.

Q 23.8 How can I get my family to leave me alone when I'm trying to work at home?

Women need to ask for their family's cooperation when they are working at home. They should advise family members to interrupt them only in an emergency and define what constitutes an "emergency." Closing the door to the workspace provides a visual signal that the worker needs privacy. Women should let their family know how long they plan to be in their office working and then honor their promise. That way, the family learns to trust that when they say they will rejoin them in two hours, they can depend on it. Home-based workers should talk to the family about work, sharing successes as well as failures and frustrations. This will help family members feel like a part of the individual's work and will increase their willingness to provide support.

Q 23.9 My nurse manager has asked me to update all of our patient education materials. What is the best way to tackle an imposing project like this?

One of the best approaches for undertaking a big project is for individuals to schedule blocks of time when they are likely to be free from interruptions. Locate a quiet place to work such as the library, a private office, or one's home. People need to consider their personal body clock and try to plan the block of time when their energy level is highest and their productivity will be enhanced. Once the place and space are established, safeguard this time by controlling all unnecessary intrusions. Limit phone calls and visitors. Divide the project into manageable sections. Set daily goals in order to complete the project within the expected timeline. Individuals can reward themselves at intervals for the progress they have made. This will sustain their motivation and interest.

Q 23.10 Even though I set aside time to work on a project, I have difficulty getting started and being productive. How can I stop myself from wasting time and spinning my wheels?

The workspace should be organized so that all needed supplies are readily available. Employees should try to eliminate any reason that would cause them to get up and leave their workspace. Plan the project ahead of time; a checklist that divides the project into small steps may help people to keep track of progress and keep their eyes on the goal. At the end of each work session, people should take a few minutes to plan their next steps so that they can pick up where they left off.

23.11   All my life, I've been a procrastinator, unable to finish projects. Am I doomed to always be this way?

A few tricks can help people avoid procrastination. People can establish the length of time they are willing to spend working on the project they have been putting off, then set a timer and discipline themselves to work consistently for that period of time (Hawke, 2002). Even if they work on a project for 15–30 minutes a day, they will be making progress. Schedule a personal reward for working hard and accomplishing a small goal. Do the unpleasant work first and get it out of the way. Otherwise, it will continue to hang over the individual's head, and she will keep finding excuses as to why she has not started to do it yet.

23.12   Are there any guidelines for conducting productive meetings to make the best use of everyone's time?

Rule number one is that a good meeting starts and ends on time. Prior to the meeting, distribute an agenda that lists discussion topics along with the individuals responsible for reporting about various issues. This allows plenty of time for participants to prepare their comments and questions. Begin the meeting by asking if there are any *new* agenda items to be added. Then establish time frames for each of the topics to ensure that all agenda items will be covered within the scheduled meeting time. The meeting leader's job is to keep the discussion on track while being attentive to the time. When discussion concludes for each topic, summarize any decisions that were made and determine both who will be responsible for any further actions and the expected date by which the action will be completed.

23.13   As a manager, all I seem to have time for is handling day-to-day crises. Can you help me find time for planning ahead for future changes?

Day-to-day crises can consume all of a manager's time and energy. If their vision is to be a *proactive* manager rather than a *reactive* manager, managers will need to regularly schedule some time for thinking about and planning for future changes. Mark time off in an appointment book (e.g., one afternoon every two weeks), and then honor it as any other commitment. Unless managers take the initiative to schedule time for planning, they will continue to be caught up in the cycle of solving daily crises rather than forging new paths into the future (Lorenz, 2005).

Q 23.14   Too many papers, too many e-mails, too many phone calls—what is the best way to deal with information overload?

Responding immediately to intrusions may seem like a good idea, but in reality it can overwhelm a person's day. Instead, set specific times during the workday to do these things. When one does pick up messages or mail, she should deal with them right then and there, if possible. Handle paper once and either file it or throw it out. It is better to take a few minutes right away to file that important paper rather than spending a half hour later trying to figure out where it might be. The same is true for e-mail messages: File them or delete them. People should file those messages that they want to retain in a folder just for that purpose; file messages that require work/answers in another folder.

Achieving a Work/Life Balance

Q 23.15   I've just started back to graduate school while also raising two kids, caring for an older adult parent, and working part time. How do I rearrange my life so that I will have enough time to read, write papers, and study?

Making room in one's life for another big commitment will mean that the person will have less time to spend on other commitments. Ask family members for their cooperation, especially regarding household chores. Emphasize that graduate school is an investment in everyone's future. Students will need to find some blocks of time for doing their schoolwork where there is quiet and where they will be free from interruptions. This time may be found at night after the children are in bed or early in the morning before everyone rises. Another option may be to stay at school after classes and go to the library to study. Students must not forget to plan their study time far enough ahead when they know there will be exams and papers due around the same time as important family occasions.

Q 23.16   **Drop-in visitors are stealing my time! Is there a way to limit these interruptions without being rude?**

People must not be afraid to close their door when they are working on an important project that needs their undivided attention. When someone arrives unexpectedly, stand up. Do not invite them to sit down. Subtly move toward the door. These actions send the message that this is not the best time for socialization. If someone suggests dropping by on a certain day, set a specific time to meet. Learn to set reasonable limits with spontaneous visitors. It is not rude for people to ask others to be respectful of their time.

Q 23.17   **After caring for patients all day long, I come home feeling exhausted. I need a nap instead of thinking about dinner and homework! What can I do to make my life easier on the home front?**

Schedule a family meeting, and set household chores for everyone. Even small children can pick up their toys before going to bed and put their dishes in the sink or their clothes in the laundry. As part of being a member of the family, everybody needs to pitch in, and when everyone does, there will be more time for play and entertainment for all. Women must recognize that they cannot do it all. Children will benefit from having these responsibilities because they will learn what it takes to run a household.

Q 23.18   **Do you have any tips for a single mom studying at home and unable to afford a sitter after school?**

Consider starting or joining a babysitting exchange group with fellow students who also have young children. This will free up some regular extended time for study. Some nurses find that they are able to study alongside their children as they do their homework. This approach gives them the opportunity to stay abreast of children's progress in school while also serving as a role model for lifelong learning. Strictly enforce an early bedtime on school nights. This will put parents' minds at ease, knowing that they will have some quiet time to study before going to bed themselves.

Q 23.19   **Any ideas for helping working mothers to feel good about their role as a mother and, at the same time, to feel that they are dependable and competent employees?**

Working mothers need to remember that they are only human. Keep the important things in focus: togetherness, education, and values. When leaving work, they must try to put their frustrations and problems aside so that they can greet their family with delight. As they travel to work, employees should place their family concerns on a back burner in order to approach their work with enthusiasm. Compromises are an intrinsic part of this dual role and will need to be made case by case. Women should let their family and employer clearly know that they are there for them, and the family and employer will, in turn, give their support. Keep things simple, and continually ask, "Will this make us happy?" If not, change may be needed.

Q 23.20   As a working mother, I know the house can't be neat and clean all the time, but I would like more order. Any suggestions?

It is difficult to have the house both neat and clean at the same time, so try to settle for one or the other. Inviting company over at intervals of approximately every three months goes a long way with helping to find time to restore order to the house. Women should set their own standards for what a clean house looks like, not the standards of their mother or mother-in-law. Most importantly, working mothers should teach those they live with that the responsibility of having a clean house rests with all family members, and everyone needs to pitch in and pick up after himself or herself.

Q 23.21   Working full time with a family, I am worried that my children will grow up feeling they didn't spend enough time with me. What are some ways to bring quality into our home life?

Quality of life is not something people can buy; they should focus their energies on what makes them happy and on cherishing the people who are meaningful to them. Make dinnertime a time for sharing the happenings of the day by turning off the television and refusing to answer the phone. Listening attentively to one's children is vitally important. Bedtime prayers, suppertime stories, and dishwashing talk can be key times to connect with one's children. Establish family rituals such as pizza on Sunday nights. Set a rule that homework is done after dinner when parents can supervise and help their children with their progress. Make a conscientious effort to attend the children's special functions as much as possible.

Q 23.22   How can I find meaning in my life again when I constantly feel pulled in so many different directions that I think I'm spinning out of control?

To find meaning in life, women need to become reacquainted with their priorities and then honor them. People *do* have a choice in how they spend their time and how they live their lives. Women should take some personal time to develop a list of their top three to five priorities. They should write them down and place the list where they will see it often. When making choices for spending their time, women must remind themselves of these priorities and ask themselves whether what they are doing fits with their life's priorities. If so, go for it! If not, they need to reflect on what choices they are making and decide whether the activity is worth doing.

Q 23.23   My life revolves around my work, and I feel out of balance. How can I revitalize myself?

High-achieving employees often spend so much time and energy invested in their work that they might neglect their family, friends, and need for leisure. Outside interests feed creativity and help employees to become even more successful than they already are. Spending long hours at work does not always mean greater productivity. Women should set the goal for themselves that they will make time for doing something other than work on a regular basis. Coming home after work may be a better ending to a hard day's work than socializing with colleagues. A key word is "balance," and people achieve this balance only by making room for *all* parts of their life (Cook et al., 2004).

Q 23.24   My days are spent doing, doing, doing for others. How can I find some time just for myself?

Look for opportunities within each day to "steal" some personal time. Lunch hour can be a source of refreshment by taking a walk outside or spending 10 minutes reading a favorite novel. An hour in the evening after the kids are in bed can be spent soaking in a bubble bath. Go to bed an hour earlier than usual and use this time for relaxing alone. If women are home with small children, they can plan their hour for while the children are napping. The hour just after lunch can be quiet time, during which children play in their rooms if they are too old to nap. If busy with carpooling, arrive for pickups early and use this time alone to journal or read. Be open to spontaneous spaces that one can use for personal renewal.

Q 23.25   With each new year, I resolve to do something on my wish list, but it never seems to happen. Do I have to wait until I retire to spend time doing something solely for me?

Individuals are in charge of their time and how they use it. Recognize that outside interests and activities help people to feel happier and more enthusiastic about life. People should identify one special thing they want to do for themselves. Then, they can look at their calendar and determine when they can plan to do it. Honor that commitment the same as any other appointment. Each individual is the only person responsible for ensuring that his or her own needs are met.

References

Cook, M.J., Strauss, B., & Noelke, N. (2004, May 11). *Time management for nurses.* Retrieved July 8, 2005, from University of Wisconsin-Madison School of Nursing online continuing education portal: http://mynursingce.son.wisc.edu/index.pl?op=show;isa=Course;iid=18330

Eckman, M., & Newman, E. (Eds.). (1997). *1,001 nursing tips and timesavers: Quick and easy tips for improving patient care* (3rd ed.). Springhouse, PA: Springhouse.

Hawke, M. (2002). There's no place like home (to work)! *Nursing Spectrum 2002 Career Fitness® Guide,* pp. 182–183.

Lorenz, J.M. (2005). Managing multiple roles. *Advance for Nurses: Serving RNs in Greater Chicago and Metro Areas of Wisconsin and Indiana, 3*(11), 16–18.

Chapter 24

Relationship Transitions

Pamela S. Dickerson, PhD, RN, BC

Friends/Colleagues

Q 24.1 **I've been a peer with my colleagues for eight years, and I've just become the nurse manager on our unit. How should I handle the change in relationship with my colleagues?**

Be honest and open with everyone. Treat each person the same as every other. The manager must be sure her actions match her words. Think carefully about things such as going out for coffee with some colleagues when not everyone is invited. Will that convey a message that the manager "likes" some people better than others? Also, be aware of the use of such possessive terms as "my nurses" or "my staff." These words may cause colleagues to perceive that the manager now sees them as "possessions" rather than people.

Q 24.2 **There are things I can share with my best friend that I wouldn't dream of sharing with my husband. Is that normal?**

Yes. Many women find that they can connect with another woman in a more empathetic way than they can with a spouse. If this helps them to feel better and be more effective in all their relationships, that is wonderful. However, if women find themselves telling "secrets" or using that friend to vent about situations involving their spouse, this may indicate that they need to rethink the purpose of the relationship.

Q 24.3 **My best friend was just diagnosed with cancer. What do I say?**

In cases like this, the words are not nearly as important as the caring message. Offering a hug and saying "I care so much about you" may be best right now. The friend with cancer may want to talk about the diagnosis and what it means to her, or she may want some quiet time alone. Friends can say, "If you would like to talk, I'm here." They might offer specific assistance, for example, driving her to physician appointments, taking her children to soccer practice, or bringing in dinner on Thursday evening. This is much more helpful than saying, "Let me know if you need anything." Anticipate the needs, and step in to provide support.

Resources are available to assist people in these challenging conversations. One example is Guilmartin's (2002) book *Healing Conversations: What to Say When You Don't Know What to Say*. Kathy's Care Cards, a line of inspirational cards introduced in 2004, may help, too. The Web site, www.kathyscarecards.com, provides examples of cards that are respectful, insightful, and heartfelt messages of support and caring. Created by a nurse, these cards originally were designed for patients with cancer but now have wider application.

Q 24.4   I had a group of close friends in college. We've lost touch as we've married, had children, established careers, or moved to other communities. I'm very sad about this. Should I do something to get the group back together?

Individuals in this situation can try to get the group together; however, not everyone in the group may feel the desire to rekindle these relationships. Remember that a person cannot control anyone else's behaviors. Set a time for a get-together, and send invitations. Those who desire a "reunion" can have a great time reminiscing; those who choose not to participate will not come. Some of the friends may respond by saying that they cannot come this time but would like to know about the next reunion. The group who attends then can decide about whether to continue getting together on a regular basis.

Significant Others/Children

Q 24.5   My partner has some habits that are driving me nuts. I'm not one for confrontation, but if a few things don't change, I'm out of here. Any suggestions?

Does the partner know what these concerns are? It is tough when both partners are not "on the same page" in terms of identifying issues and solutions. Many people are fearful of "confrontation" because they see it as negative and blaming. Refocus that thinking—look at confrontation as a way to identify issues and together develop strategies to deal with those issues. For example, instead of, "If you leave the lid off the toothpaste again, I'm going to squeeze it all over you," try, "I work really hard to keep the bathroom clean, and when I see the lid off the toothpaste I feel like there's just more work for me." The individual has confronted the issue, not blamed the partner. Now one of the partners has opened the door to talking about how to resolve this situation in a way that is agreeable to both of them.

Q 24.6 **My partner loves violent and "X-rated" movies, fast-food dinners, and outdoor activities. I prefer a quiet dinner and an evening at a play or opera. I find that I typically go along with what my partner wants to do, then feel frustrated and angry that my needs are not considered. How can I deal with this?**

Partners need to be very careful about losing themselves in the relationship. In a caring, sharing relationship, both partners' needs are acknowledged and addressed. This might be done in a variety of ways. Maybe the partners alternate weekends—one weekend at the movies, the next at a play. Perhaps they decide that each of them will have one evening a week to do an independent activity. In any case, failure to meet one's own needs may lead to depression, loss of self-esteem, resentment, anger, or other negative consequences. A resource such as Lerner's (2001) book *The Dance of Connection* might give partners some suggestions for effective ways to communicate their concerns and advocate for their own needs.

Q 24.7 **My 13-year-old daughter is driving me nuts. Between her menarche hormones and my perimenopausal hormones, we spend a lot of time butting heads. Any suggestions?**

The mother in this case has made a good beginning by recognizing that much of the behavior she is seeing is hormone driven. Teens can cause a lot of family stress as they struggle to define their own identities. The biggest things the mother can do right now are (a) continue to express, through both words and actions, her unconditional love for her daughter, (b) establish and maintain limits for acceptable and unacceptable behaviors, and (c) take care of herself so that she has the energy and patience to help her daughter with her needs.

Q 24.8 **My relationship with my partner has been increasingly difficult to maintain. I've told him I would leave if things didn't change, but I haven't seen any difference. What can I do?**

Be very careful about sending mixed messages. This person's words are saying she will take action, but her actions are saying she is going to continue things the way they are. Empty threats very quickly lose their punch. Identify the specific issues of concern, and address those. It may be helpful for one or both partners to work with a counselor to do this. Making threats is not effective. However, one may establish consequences. In other words, state that "if 'x' does not happen within three months, I will leave." The important thing is to be consistent—if a partner says she is going to leave, she should be prepared to do so.

Q 24.9 **My partner and I have decided to separate after 14 years together. There's no major catastrophe; it seems like we've just grown apart. I feel like I've failed, though. What did I do wrong?**

It is very likely that this partner did nothing wrong. Women often feel a sense of failure if life is not perfect. Women think it is their job to "fix" things, and they want life to flow smoothly. If the partners have tried addressing their differences, communicating their concerns, and perhaps seeking counseling, all to no avail, it might be time to let go of the relationship. The partner should do a thorough self-inventory of her feelings. It is okay to feel sad and to go through the stages of grief and loss. Be sure to separate *grief* from *guilt*. Grieving is a healthy process with a goal of resolution of the sad experience. Guilt, however, leads to negative behaviors of blaming self or others. There is no positive outcome to guilt.

Q 24.10 **We have a "yours, mine, and ours" blended family. How do I help the children to get along with each other?**

Children in this situation often feel torn by divided loyalties. Their primary allegiance is to the birth parent, but they believe (or are told) that they should love the parent-by-marriage and the other child/children. Both parents can help by providing equal time, attention, and support to each child and creating a home where each child can interact with parents and siblings in a caring manner. Remember that parents cannot "buy" a child's love or loyalty or "make" this happen. Time and positive experiences will help.

Q24.11 **I am getting a divorce. I have three children, ages 2, 6, and 10. How do I help them deal with this?**

The two-year-old will not be able to understand the issues but will pick up the sense of unease in the household. This may result in behavior change or an increase in self-comforting behavior like thumb-sucking. The 6- and 10-year-olds will be more aware of the specific issues and will understand basic explanations. Children often perceive themselves as the cause of disruption in families. They need to know that they are not the cause of the divorce and that both parents will continue to love and care about them (if this is indeed the case). Check with a children's librarian at the local library; a number of books have been written for children to help them deal with divorce.

Q24.12 **I've just learned that I'm going to become a grandmother. What changes should I anticipate?**

Congratulations! Becoming a grandparent is a major milestone. Be prepared to enjoy it. A bumper sticker exists that reads, "If I'd known grandparenting was this much fun, I would have done it first."

People may perceive the arrival of their first grandchild as an indication of their own aging. They may need to think through their own feelings before they are ready to welcome the grandchild.

Each age and stage of development brings its own challenges and rewards. It is important to take the time to appreciate and enjoy.

Q24.13 **My daughter got very angry with me when she thought I didn't like her fiancé. They eloped, and she left me a note saying that she will never talk to me again. I'm devastated. What can I do?**

Nothing, right now. As time goes by, the intensity of the pain will diminish. It is important for the mother to accept that she cannot control her daughter's behavior. If she knows where the daughter is, the mother can call or write her a letter affirming her love for her and stating that she will open her heart and her home to her when the daughter is ready to resume contact (if the mother does, in fact, feel that way). Using the letter or phone call to blame, argue, or defend will not help. The mother should keep her expectations minimal so that she will not be disappointed by not getting a response. The mother must not blame herself for her daughter's actions.

Q 24.14 I find myself as a grandmother having just assumed "parenting" responsibilities for my grandchildren. What should I be aware of?

First, clarify what this means. Is the grandmother caring for the grandchildren while the parents work or are traveling, because the parents are not doing the parenting, or because the parents are ill or deceased?

Several key issues need to be kept in mind. The grandparent should be sure that she has legally designated guardianship or a permission slip signed by the parents allowing her to authorize medical care for the children, if necessary. Written authorization also will be important if she is picking up children from school or childcare facilities.

If the children's parents are still in the picture, grandparents need to be sure that they have a clear understanding about who has responsibility for things such as discipline, daily schedules, and education. Once those decisions have been made, they should be implemented consistently. Keep lines of communication open, and reinforce to the children that they are loved and cared for. AARP (www.aarp.org/ families) has a number of resources available for grandparents who have active parenting responsibilities for their grandchildren.

Q 24.15 For many years, my focus has been my partner and my children. I'm at a point in my life now where I would like my focus to be me. How can I make that happen?

First, women can make a conscious decision to put themselves first. Women often give lip service to self-care, but they direct their energies toward meeting the needs of others. One tenet of the American Nurses Association's (2001) Code of Ethics stated that nurses owe the same duty to themselves as to others. If they do not nurture themselves, they soon run out of energy to provide care for others. Just as women focus on meeting the needs of others, they need to thoughtfully consider how they are meeting their own needs. That is not selfish; it is survival.

Women need to think carefully about their behaviors and choices. They must give themselves permission to live their dreams—decide what they want to do, make a plan, and make it happen!

Aging Parents

Q 24.16 **My parents are getting older. They live 200 miles away. I don't think they are taking very good care of themselves and their home. Is it appropriate to move them here so I can keep an eye on them?**

That is a real dilemma. It is natural for people to be concerned about their aging parents and to want them to be safe and healthy. However, unless a person's parents have a form of dementia or are otherwise incapable of making their own decisions, it is inappropriate to start making decisions for them.

Many older adults prefer to stay in their own communities with their families, friends, places of worship, grocery stores, libraries, and healthcare providers. If parents choose this option, the children can help them look for support and assistance resources in their home community.

If children think their parents would be interested in relocating, they should explore the pros and cons with them. Help them in the decision-making process, including assessment of resources and choices regarding types of living arrangements, geographic preferences, and logistic concerns, such as what furniture and belongings to keep or sell.

Q 24.17 **My parents are in their 80s. We need to talk about things such as wills, finances, and funeral and burial preferences. How do I initiate these discussions?**

Talking about death and dying is difficult for many people. It is important, however, to talk about these issues, and the sooner the better.

When the time comes for implementation of the plans, the spouse or child must make important decisions in a stressful situation. The more clearly people have explained and documented their wishes, the easier it is for those who need to make decisions on their behalf. A good resource to guide people with helpful discussion points and suggestions is the book *Talking About Death Won't Kill You* by Virginia Morris (2001). This and similar books are available in public libraries or bookstores.

Having these discussions with one's parents may open the door for the adult child to talk about her own wishes with her partner and her children. People do not have to wait until they are "old" to talk about and plan for their end-of-life wishes. States have different requirements regarding legal documents; be sure to check and follow these requirements.

Q 24.18   My father just died. I find myself wandering down the street, wondering how people can go on about their work and their lives when my life has just turned upside down. Is this normal?

Yes. After a death or traumatic experience, it is normal to spend a few days in a "bubble." People need to allow themselves this time to process what has happened and begin to deal with their grief and loss.

Q 24.19   I remember being sad and a little out-of-sorts when my father died. But now that my mother has just died, I feel really overwhelmed. Why is this so different?

A tremendous difference exists between the death of the first parent and the death of the second. When the first parent dies, the child still has a parent-child relationship with the surviving parent. When the second parent dies, the child becomes an orphan. This is very hard.

Additional decisions and tasks are present, too, when the second parent dies. What does the child do with the house? The furniture? The photo albums? The jewelry? How does one probate a will? Serve as an executor? File final tax returns?

Death of the second parent also causes the child to think about her own mortality. Especially if she is an only child or the oldest child, she is now the oldest generation of her family. Thinking about this on an intellectual level is very different than dealing with the reality on an emotional level.

References

American Nurses Association. (2001). *Code of ethics with interpretive statements.* Washington, DC: Author.

Guilmartin, N. (2002). *Healing conversations: What to say when you don't know what to say.* San Francisco: Jossey-Bass.

Lerner, H. (2001). *The dance of connection: How to talk to someone when you're mad, hurt, scared, frustrated, insulted, or desperate.* New York: HarperCollins.

Morris, V. (2001). *Talking about death won't kill you.* New York: Workman.

Resources

AARP: www.aarp.org
Kathy's Care Cards: www.kathyscarecards.com

Chapter 25
Surviving Menopause

Leona Lipari Lee, MA, RN

Background

Q 25.1 **I'm only 42 years old, and I'm starting to have hot flashes. I can't possibly be in menopause already, can I?**

Yes. It is very possible that this woman is experiencing perimenopause, the period of 5–10 years surrounding menopause. During perimenopause, which can begin when women are in their mid-30s but more typically occurs from mid-40s to mid-50s, women may experience hot flashes and irregular periods, among other symptoms.

Q 25.2 **What exactly is menopause, and how will I know when I'm there?**

Perimenopause is a process that occurs over a period of years, including the time of cessation of a woman's periods. Perimenopause occurs as the ovaries gradually stop functioning and hormone levels drop. Once hormone levels have stabilized, women can expect some relief from the symptoms of perimenopause, such as menstrual irregularity, hot flashes, insomnia, and mood swings. Menopause is said to have occurred when a woman has had no menses for one year.

Signs and Symptoms

Q 25.3 **What are some of the physical and emotional things that might happen to me during the perimenopause period?**

Besides the most common symptoms mentioned previously—hot flashes, insomnia, irregular menstrual cycles with heavier and/or lighter flow—some women experience vaginal dryness, vaginal and urinary tract infections, headaches, and muscle pain. Other symptoms, more emotional in nature, also may occur. These might include mood swings, anxiety attacks, lack of concentration, and moodiness.

Q 25.4   My doctor tells me I need a total hysterectomy with removal of both ovaries and my uterus. My friend said I'm going to feel like I'm going through menopause. Is this true?

The friend is correct. Removal of the ovaries as part of a total hysterectomy will cause women to experience the symptoms of menopause because they will have a sudden drop in estrogen and progesterone levels. Even if menopause is the result of surgery, women still might be at risk for physical problems often associated with natural menopause, such as heart disease and osteoporosis.

Q 25.5   What causes these embarrassing hot flashes?

Hot flashes are the result of a drop in levels of estrogen, changes in the brain, and dilation of blood vessels. Some experts believe that low estrogen levels cause the brain's hypothalamus, which regulates body temperature, to trigger the dilation of blood vessels in the skin. This results in the hot flash.

Q 25.6   How do I stay cool when I'm in the throes of a hot flash?

Women can do several things to keep themselves cool. Wear light, nonsynthetic clothing. Stay away from spicy foods, hot baths, hot rooms, warm beds, hot anything. Do not overexercise or get overheated. Avoid hot beverages and alcohol. Cool down by turning up the air conditioning. Sip cool beverages. Women can fan themselves and should try to avoid stress.

Q 25.7   I'm so moody that my family can't stand to be around me. What can I do?

Women need to recognize that their ups and downs are related to the fluctuating levels of hormones in their body. They should discuss with their healthcare provider whether the use of hormone replacement therapy (HRT), at least on a short-term basis, might be helpful. Exercise is probably one of the most beneficial things women can do to fight moodiness. Eat healthy foods, and avoid sugar, caffeine, and alcohol. Some recommend vitamin B supplements. In certain cases, other types of medications besides hormones have been found to be helpful in relieving both moodiness and hot flashes. Women should check with their healthcare provider and take care of their bodies. Try new makeup, new interests, a new self.

Q 25.8   I'm really depressed. Can menopause be causing this?

Most definitely. Menopause can cause menopausal blues, typically of short duration. However, women need to understand the difference between menopausal blues and clinical depression. If their sadness is accompanied by prolonged feelings of hopelessness, slowed body movements and speech, sleeping all the time or having difficulty sleeping, and thoughts of suicide, they must seek medical attention.

Q 25.9   I wake up with night sweats. Is there any help for the insomnia that has plagued me since I started menopause?

Several things can help menopausal women get a good night's sleep. Go to bed at the same time every night. If women cannot fall asleep after 10–20 minutes or if they awaken after being asleep, they should get up and do something relaxing. Exercise early in the evening, take a warm bath, and have a snack before bedtime. Most importantly, keep the bedroom temperature cool.

Q 25.10   Are anxiety and panic attacks associated with menopause?

Very often, women will begin experiencing anxiety during perimenopause. This sometimes happens because of decreased estrogen, which leads to decreased production of endorphins (brain chemicals that enhance a person's well-being). This lack of estrogen and subsequent reduced endorphin level causes women to be less calm and more anxious. Also, increased adrenalin during an actual hot flash may be responsible for varying levels of anxiety and panic.

Q 25.11   I'm so tired lately and very irritable. What's happening to me?

Feeling tired and irritable are common signs of menopause. If women are taking a progesterone product, they may find themselves to be more irritable. Lack of sleep also contributes to feeling both tired and irritable.

Q 25.12   The worst thing about menopause for me is that I can't concentrate, and I'm really forgetful. What can I do about it?

To regain their concentration, menopausal women need to practice focusing. Try to get a good night's sleep. Remember to keep a sense of humor about forgetting and misplacing things. Although it is important to rule out other potential causes of one's loss of concentration, it is quite possible that this, too, shall pass.

Q 25.13   Does menopause cause you to lose your sexual drive?

The decrease in sexual desire that women may experience occurs because of the dryness and tightness of the vagina. It is hard for a woman to feel sexy when she is uncomfortable. These problems are associated with estrogen decline, and locally applied preparations may relieve them. Women should check with their healthcare provider to see what might be helpful for them.

Q 25.14   The weirdest thing happened to me the other day. I felt like my skin was crawling. Surely this doesn't have anything to do with menopause?

This symptom, called formication, has been linked to menopause and may be caused by estrogen deprivation. When a woman feels as though she has insects crawling under her skin, she should not panic. This is a temporary phenomenon usually appearing 12–24 months after the last menstrual period. The episodes last only a few moments and usually disappear on their own. Some people have found taking estrogen to be helpful.

Q 25.15   I thought menopause means your period stops. Why are my periods heavier?

During perimenopause, women's levels of estrogen fluctuate. Not only may they experience heavier periods, but also their periods might become extremely irregular. Some women experience more frequent periods instead of monthly, sometimes lighter periods, sometimes heavier. They may even skip a month or two. Menstrual irregularity is very common during perimenopause. Note that it *is* still possible for women to get pregnant as long as they are ovulating, so birth control practices during this time are a good idea.

Interventions

Q 25.16   I'm really nervous about taking HRT. What should I do?

Women must weigh all the pros and cons and then discuss their options with a knowledgeable healthcare provider. Recent research, as part of the Women's Health Initiative (National Institutes of Health, 2004), showed a slight but significant increased risk for breast cancer and heart disease when taking continuous estrogen/progestin therapy at a specific dosage level. Many specific drugs are available for osteoporosis and heart disease. Some physicians are prescribing short-term HRT to prevent hot flashes and the emotional component of menopause but are not advocating long-term use of HRT. Research shows that more than half of the women who discontinued HRT saw a return of symptoms, so women will need to stay informed ("HRT May Postpone, Not Prevent, Menopausal Symptoms," 2005).

Q 25.17   What are some other things I can do to get through perimenopause?

Practice good nutrition by eating lots of fruits and vegetables. Some people consider adding vitamin and mineral supplements, especially calcium and vitamin D. Exercise, using both aerobic and weight-bearing activities. Women can take care of their appearance and use stress-reducing strategies.

Q 25.18   I won't go crazy, will I?

Women experiencing perimenopause will not go crazy, although they may feel like they are at times. Remember, perimenopause will not last forever! Please note that women who are experiencing symptoms of severe depression or having suicidal thoughts must contact a mental health center or their healthcare provider for support and assistance during this time.

Postmenopausal Characteristics

Q 25.19   When will perimenopause be over?

Although women may feel as though it will never be over, they will make it to the other side of perimenopause. For some women, the whole process may take as long as 10 years, whereas for others, just a couple. For the lucky ones, the symptoms never appear—one day, no period. Most women will experience one or more of the symptoms discussed in this chapter in the time surrounding the last menstrual period. All women will make it to the other side of perimenopause, unless something unrelated to menopause gets them first!

Q 25.20   After menopause, will I feel like my old self again?

No, women will not feel like their old selves after menopause. Life will be different. They actually can feel better. Lots of things happen as women go through menopause that may change them forever. If one's children leave home to go to college, think about joining them (at a different school, perhaps). Use the changes to foster personal improvement. A woman can look at her own life goals—what can she do to achieve them? What can she do for *herself*? This is an important time to enjoy life!

Q 25.21   What happens after menopause? Will I feel old?

Postmenopausal women may find a renewed sense of energy and purpose. If they do not, they should work to acquire one. Suggestions include joining clubs, meeting new people, or going back to school.

Q 25.22   Will I be at a greater risk for health problems after menopause?

Yes. Osteoporosis is a major problem in the postmenopausal period, and so is heart disease. But women can do things to prevent both. Exercise and take calcium and vitamin D if indicated to help to prevent osteoporosis. Exercise and healthy living also help to prevent heart disease. Women should consult with their healthcare provider to explore their personal risk factors and see whether other interventions might be appropriate for them.

Q 25.23   How can I achieve good emotional and physical health once I'm beyond menopause?

Women can decide that they are going to make it through menopause and be better than ever. Then review this chapter and others in the book to help to develop a personal action plan. Reach for the stars!

References

HRT may postpone, not prevent, menopausal symptoms. (2005, Fall/Winter). *Penn Ob/Gyn Care Newsletter.* Retrieved July 13, 2005, from http://www.pennhealth.com/obgyn/news/05fall/hrt.html

National Institutes of Health. (2004, March). *Medical encyclopedia: Hormone replacement therapy (HRT)*. Retrieved July 13, 2005, from http://www.nlm.nih.gov/medlineplus/ency/article/007111.htm

Resources

Lee, L.L. (2002). *How to survive menopause without going crazy* (Rev. ed.). San Jose, CA: Authors Choice Press.

North American Menopause Society: www.menopause.org/default.htm

Sheehy, G. (1998). *The silent passage* (Rev. ed.). New York: Random House.

Chapter 26

Adult Children and Aging Parents

Lynn Dobb, MA, and Lisa Durham, MSW, LISW

Background

26.1 Is it true that we "parent" our parents as they get older?

No. Although adults may become more involved in their parents' care and day-to-day needs, it is crucial to remember that their parents are always their parents. Regardless of their physical or cognitive needs, the parents are still their elders and have a lifetime of experiences greater than theirs. Although the relationship may change, they will forever be their parents.

26.2 Do we all lose our memory as we get older?

Most definitely no! Although minor memory loss occurs with aging, significant memory loss is not a normal part of aging. If memory loss impairs one's ability to function daily, he or she needs to be evaluated by a specialist. Someone might exhibit memory loss for many reasons, some of which may be reversible. A complete medical evaluation definitely is in order if memory loss is a concern. Examples of reversible memory loss, if properly diagnosed and treated, include side effects from common medications, depression, nutritional or metabolic disorders, and cardiovascular or infectious diseases, as well as several others. Clearly, not all memory loss indicates Alzheimer disease. It is a myth to think that memory loss and confusion are a part of aging. The majority of older adults remain alert and able. A slower speed of recall and a natural decrease in retention of noncritical information are a normal part of aging. The analogy of a filing cabinet often has been used when thinking of retrieval of information from an older person's brain. The older adult has many more files stored in his or her "filing cabinet" than a younger person. It just takes a little longer to retrieve the right file!

26.3   Where do I find a "good" doctor who understands older adult health issues?

Ideally, if people can find one in their community or within reasonable driving distance, they should seek out the care of a geriatrician. Board-certified geriatricians specialize in the diagnosis, treatment, and prevention of disorders in older people. People can call their local Area Agency on Aging for resources available in their community. If a geriatrician is not available in one's community, then an internist or family physician that serves older adults could be an option. Talk with people in the medical community, and ask for a recommendation. It also may be possible to make an appointment to sit down and talk with a physician to essentially "screen" for compatibility. People should explain their health issues and get a sense of how the physician would treat or respond to their concerns. Patients need to trust their gut and should not hesitate to "shop" around. The doctor-patient relationship is one of the most important relationships a person will ever establish.

26.4   How do I get my parents to be willing to accept help, and where do I start?

This is a very difficult question. Admitting that one needs help meeting his or her own needs is very difficult, and all people do it on their own timeline. It is frustrating for someone to watch his or her parents refuse help and have their needs go unmet or under-met. No magic answer exists, but here are a few suggestions.
- Educate them on available services and the costs.
- Get someone outside the family to talk to them about accepting help, for example, a pastor, priest, rabbi, family friend, neighbor, social worker, or nurse.
- If parents are relying on adult children to fulfill their needs, and the children are overwhelmed, they need to set limits and stick to them. This is much easier said than done. By setting limits, children are not saying that they are not going to do something that their parents need to be done. However, it is important for the children to let their parents know there are other ways to get these needs met, and they will help their parents to explore and arrange for outside assistance.
- Continue to educate them, again and again.
- If and when a crisis happens, be there with the information and support to get the necessary services in place.

The Area Agency on Aging, the local Office on Aging, and the hospital, if the parent is an inpatient, are good places to start. Locate these services through the Eldercare Locator at 800-677-1116.

26.5 **Do my parents have to lose all of their assets before they can get help with homecare costs?**

No. Many programs exist to help to defray the costs of homecare services, such as Meals-on-Wheels, transportation programs, homemaker services, and others. Some of these programs operate on a donation basis, some are on a sliding-fee scale, and others may involve qualifying for Medicaid. Every state differs regarding eligibility and availability of programs. All of these services can be purchased privately. However, proper planning and input from the right professionals can save people time, frustration, and money. A financial planner, estate planner, or an elder law attorney can help people determine the best way to plan for home care or long-term care services.

Caregiver Challenges

26.6 **Is it okay for my aging parents to move in with my husband, our teens, and me?**

Adult children may face the dilemma of helping their parents to find housing that also provides support, safety, and care. Sometimes having their parents move into their home is a viable option; sometimes it is not. Before taking such a step, the children must consider several issues:

- What do the parents want? Do they want to live with my family? As adult children, it is sometimes easy for them to forget to ask their parents what they want. They get so fixated on solving the problem that their parents' wishes often become secondary, if noticed at all.
- What is their relationship with the parents like now? Do the child and parents get along? Has there always been an underlying tension there? Do the parents like their child's spouse?

Although these questions may be easy to minimize, the answers to them are vital indicators of whether moving one's parents into his or her home will succeed. Recognize that in becoming a caregiver for one's parents, the relationship will change. Parents and adult children who have good relationships are much more likely to have a successful living arrangement than those who have had problems in the past. Although this option may seem the easiest choice today, in the long run, it may be the hardest one.

Q 26.7   I'm missing work to care for my mother. I can't keep on doing this. Who can help me?

Many caregivers rely on adult day services to provide care for their family member so that they can continue to work. To access this service, contact the local Area Agency on Aging or Office on Aging. This office can assist with linking caregivers to other ongoing services to provide intermittent care for their parent. Some states are starting to experiment with paying family members to care for their loved one. People should check with their Area Agency on Aging to see whether their state is one of them. The National Family Caregiver Support Program may be able to help caregivers as well. In addition, the Alzheimer's Association has many programs and educational opportunities for family members caring for someone with a memory disorder.

Q 26.8   My siblings and I are doing the best we can, but we're stressed out. What's out there to help us to figure out what we should do?

The good news is that professionals are available to help caregivers with options. The Area Agency on Aging, the local Office on Aging, the Alzheimer's Association, or a local aging services provider is an excellent place to start. The Internet has a wealth of wonderful Web sites with information on available resources. The National Family Caregiver Support Program, a program of the Older Americans Act, is designed to help people find the information, assistance, counseling, services, and education they need to address their family's needs. People can access this program through their local Area Agency on Aging. This agency also can help family caregivers find a support group to learn from others in similar situations.

Q 26.9   I feel as if I'm doing all the work and my brother just flies in for an occasional weekend to visit Mom and Dad. My parents think he walks on water, and I'm busting my chops trying to help them every day. This makes me angry. What should I do?

This is a very common scenario. It is so difficult for the local child to measure up to the out-of-towner, and it is difficult for the out-of-town child to feel as though he or she has contributed to the parents' care. The best thing for siblings to do is to have an honest discussion about their feelings, without blaming the other sibling. This can be a daunting task and may need to be facilitated by an outside party, such as a social worker, geriatric care manager (GCM), or someone from the sibling's faith community. The conversation should include things that the long-distance sibling could do to help the local sibling with caregiving. For example, when the sibling visits, take the opportunity to take a vacation or a respite from providing care. Perhaps the sibling can contribute financially to care so that the other is not entirely responsible. Remember that this needs to be an ongoing conversation, and one that should include the siblings' parents.

26.10   **What can I do to help care for my parents, who live in another state? How do I find out what is available where they live?**

The best place to start to learn what services and programs are available for one's parents would be to call the Eldercare Locator (800-677-1116). Children also can go online to www.eldercare.gov. This resource gives callers access to an extensive network of state and local organizations that serve older people anywhere in the United States. The Eldercare Locator will help the caller to identify the most appropriate organization for information and assistance in an older person's community. Hours of operation are 9 am–8 pm eastern standard time. Children will need to know the county in which the parent is living.

Older Adult Care Options and Services

26.11   **What is a geriatric care manager?**

GCMs are professionals who use multiple skills to provide assistance and support to older adults. They can represent the adult children who live or work in another state and have limited time to travel to manage their parents' or relatives' affairs. It is wise to look for a social worker, nurse, counselor, or other healthcare professional with extensive knowledge of community resources and government programs for older adults. Certification as a GCM is a recently recommended requirement but not a mandated requirement. If relatives decide to hire a GCM or other healthcare professional, they may want to contact the National Association of Professional Geriatric Care Managers. Its Web site, www.caremanager.org, is an excellent starting point. A checklist of questions to ask GCMs is available in Ellen F. Rubenson's (2000) book *When Aging Parents Can't Live Alone.*

Q 26.12   What kinds of housing options exist for my aging parents?

A continuum of housing options exists for older adults in the United States today. From living in their own home with services, to a senior apartment facility, to a continuous care community (which includes assisted living), older adults have more choices than ever. Only when beginning to look at cost does one realize that these options are not for everyone. These options include the following.

- **Senior independent apartments:** These apartments often are designed for older adults who still are able to meet most of their own needs but would enjoy the safety, security, and low maintenance of an apartment. Some of these apartments may be federally subsidized, limiting rent to 30% of the older adult's adjusted income. Others may be independent, not-for-profit, or for-profit apartment complexes.

- **Assisted living:** Assisted living varies greatly from state to state. No single accepted national definition exists. However, the American Association of Homes and Services for the Aging (AAHSA, 2005) defines assisted living as a program that provides and/or arranges for daily meals, personal and other supportive services, health care, and 24-hour oversight to people residing in a group residential facility who need assistance with the activities of daily living. Often, assisted living is described as a *philosophy* of services that maximizes each resident's independence and dignity. Some states have Medicaid-supported assisted living to help with the cost.

- **Continuing care retirement communities (CCRCs):** CCRCs provide a continuum of housing and service options. From independent living, to assisted living, to the nursing home, these communities are campuses that allow the resident to stay within that community as care needs change. CCRCs also provide a contract for care so that the person is guaranteed housing and services within the community for the rest of his or her life. For more information, the Continuing Care Accreditation Commission (www.carf.org/aging) offers pamphlets on CCRCs.

- **Nursing homes, or nursing facilities:** Nursing homes are facilities that provide 24-hour supervision and nursing care for residents who are no longer able to care for themselves, with or without assistance from families. Designed with a medical model, many nursing homes have semiprivate rooms, with a nurse's station centrally located. An individual must meet a certain "level of care" to be eligible for nursing home care.

Medicare does not pay for long-term placement in a nursing home. It will cover the cost of a rehabilitative stay; for example, if a person is recovering from a stroke or a hip fracture. Medicare will pay only for the rehabilitation stay, anywhere from two to eight weeks, depending on the nature of the admission and the person's progress. If, after that time, the person believes he or she needs to remain in the nursing home, then the patient must pay privately or apply for Medicaid. A wonderful resource for more information is the AAHSA, a nonprofit organization, at www.aahsa.org.

26.13   What kinds of services are available to older adults who want to live in their own homes, and how do you pay for them?

Many services are available to older adults in the community. The following descriptions are services that are consistent among states.
- **Adult day care, or adult day service:** A facility that provides supervision, activities, meals, and interaction for older adults who need care, supervision, or socialization during the day hours. This service is invaluable to caregivers who need to continue to work. They can drop their loved one off prior to work or have them picked up by a van and then returned at the end of the day. This service also is available for respite, so that nonworking caregivers can get a break, run errands, or meet their own needs. These centers vary in the types of additional services they might provide, such as bathing and personal care, or occupational or physical therapy.
- **Emergency response system:** A necklace or pendant that can be worn by a person who is alone, has multiple health issues, or is fearful of falling. Upon pushing a button, the wearer can access emergency assistance.
- **Homemaker services:** Assistance with general housecleaning, laundry, grocery shopping, and errands
- **Meals-on-Wheels, or home-delivered meals:** Meals that are brought to the individual's home on a daily basis to meet nutritional needs
- **Personal care services:** Assistance with bathing, dressing, mobility, and grooming
- **Transportation:** Generally available for medical appointments but also for therapy or lab appointments, as well as other errands if availability permits

The costs of each of these services vary greatly from state to state and community to community. All services are available via private pay. Funding under Title III of the Older Americans Act also provides limited coverage for these services. States may have Medicaid waiver programs that pay for a combination of services, as well as provide case management to assess, arrange for, and monitor service provision. Many states have their own aging services delivery systems that supplement the costs of these services. People should start with their Area Agency on Aging to determine the availability and eligibility of these services for them. They also may contact the county Office on Aging or their local aging services provider as a starting point. People can find these via the Eldercare Locator.

Q 26.14   Where can I find affordable medications for my parents?

The Medicare Prescription Drug Benefit became available in January 2006. It is a possible benefit for every Medicare beneficiary, and everyone should explore it. As this is a comprehensive change in the Medicare program, much is not yet known. The best plan of action is for people to explore the different programs and benefits available in their area and determine which plan, if any, is right for them. Some beneficiaries may have better coverage through their retirement plan. Many online resources exist to assist people in this process, the primary one being www.medicare.gov. People can contact their state's Senior Health Insurance Program, or SHIP, to have access to volunteers to help them to understand this new benefit.

In addition, each state and local community is attempting to provide assistance in some way. Some of these programs may change as a result of the Medicare Prescription Drug Program, but here is a current description of some of these resources for patients.

• Patients should ask the physician for samples; many times, physicians do not offer this unless they realize there is a financial need.
• Many manufacturers have patient assistance programs that allow patients to apply for free medications; each manufacturer has different eligibility requirements, and not all medications are covered.
• Some drug manufacturers offer their own discount drug cards.
• Patients should check to see whether their state has a discount drug program or a discount card.
• People also can contact their local aging agency to see whether it maintains a list of local, state, and national programs.

Q 26.15   What is respite care?

"Respite care" refers to short-term assistance for people who care for older adults in their homes. It is a break from caregiving so that caregivers can have some time to run errands, go out to dinner, or just have some uninterrupted rest. Trained professionals or volunteers care for the older person for short periods in the home. A facility that provides 24-hour care can provide a longer period of respite care so that caregivers can have a break or go out of town. Fees vary depending on the location and duration of respite.

26.16 **Does Medicare cover the cost of long-term care? What exactly is long-term care?**

Medicare pays for *very limited, short-term* assistance for care, based on need for skilled care prescribed by a physician. Medicare is not responsible for the cost of long-term care in the home or the nursing home, nor does it currently cover the cost of assisted living.

The definition of long-term care has changed over the years. Although it used to be identified as mostly nursing home care, it now is viewed as a continuum of housing and service options that assist older adults and disabled people to live as independently as possible, where and how they choose. It covers all combinations of housing, from one's own home, to the home of a relative, to assisted living, to CCRCs, to nursing facilities. It also includes services that assist the individual and family caregivers. These services include home-delivered meals, assistance with housekeeping, grocery shopping, transportation, adult day care, personal care, and assistance with bill paying and applying for benefits.

End-of-Life Issues

26.17 **What are advance directives? Why should I worry about them? How do I get them?**

End-of-life issues have become much more complicated over the years. Medical advances have presented many choices to older people and their families. The array of choices and decisions often is overwhelming and confusing. People of all ages are haunted by the image of a prolonged, painful end of life. Respecting a loved one's wishes can be done if advance directives are in place. Specifically, advance directives are documents that serve as an opportunity for an older person, or any individual for that matter, to discuss end-of-life choices.

- **Directives for health care:** Typically, two types of legal documents exist to indicate a person's instructions for end-of-life health care.

One type outlines the kind of medical attention desired, whereas the other names another person who can make sure these wishes are carried out. The names of these legal documents may vary from state to state, so people should be sure to check for the terms used in their state.

- **Durable power of attorney for health care:** A person designates another (an "agent" or "proxy") to make healthcare decisions in the event the person becomes incapacitated or unable to communicate.
- **Living will:** This document details a person's wishes about medical care at the end of his or her life in the event that the person becomes incapacitated and is unable to provide instructions. The living will usually directs that comfort should be maintained while illness takes a natural course.
- **Do-not-resuscitate order:** This physician order instructs medical personnel not to use cardiopulmonary resuscitation if the person's heart stops beating.

Many advantages exist to having directives in writing prior to a crisis event. Clearly, if these are created, people can have greater comfort in knowing that their wishes will be honored. The directives can be flexible and tailored to an individual's wishes. Advance directives can be revoked at any time as long as the person is mentally competent. Forms for advance healthcare directives vary from state to state and are available from most hospitals, nursing homes, or legal aid associations.

Q 26.18   What key documents should I be aware of that my parents might have?

Although it may feel awkward, it is in both parents' *and* adult children's best interest to discuss and share some critical information on end-of-life issues and general financial and medical information. In the event that adult children need this information and their parents are not available to access it for them, a written list of important information will be incredibly helpful to have during an already stressful time. Several tools exist to help to organize this information. The personal profile (Ohio State University Extension [OSUE], 2002) is one such tool that was developed by the Senior Series collaborative team of OSUE agents and professionals from Ohio in the field of aging. The personal profile tool is available for free at OSUE's Ohioline Web site at www.ohioline.osu.edu/ss-fact/0169.html.

The following are examples of the information that would be helpful to have on hand or to know where to access.

- List of doctors' names, addresses, and phone numbers
- Names and addresses of the financial planner, executor of the will, funeral director, insurance agent, person with the power of attorney, durable power of attorney for health care, and tax person
- Names and phone numbers of neighbors to contact in case of an emergency
- Professional addresses of the local bank, place of worship, hospital, funeral home, and insurance agency
- Document information such as income tax records, citizenship papers, deeds to cemetery plots or property, driver's licenses, advance directives, insurance policies (car, health, accident, and house), Medicare and Medicaid information, mortgage or loan documents, Social Security information, and marriage certificates.
- Titles—car, house, boat, other
- Vehicle registrations—car, boat, other
- Financial information—bank accounts, safety deposit box, credit cards, retirement accounts, other
- Personal choice information—organ donation, burial decisions, funeral services, memorial, wake, cremation, other

State and Federal Programs

26.19   Does every state offer the same services for older adults?

Yes and no. Every state has a state unit or department of aging and is divided into planning and service areas with their own Area Agencies on Aging. Theoretically, the federal government has set up a system for accessing services in a uniform fashion across the country. However, some parts of the country or even parts of one state have more services than another. Some communities have passed local levies that are dedicated to providing services to seniors to promote independence and the option to "age in place." Communities with local levies tend to be more "service rich" as a result of additional dollars for programs to assist seniors in the community. To learn more about the services available in their community, people can contact their local Area Agency on Aging.

26.20   What is an Area Agency on Aging?

The federal government mandated Area Agencies on Aging under the Older Americans Act, which was originally passed in 1965. This act created the Administration on Aging (AoA) under the U.S. Department of Health and Human Services. The AoA created 10 regional Offices on Aging and then 57 state units on aging. The 670 Area Agencies on Aging fall under the state units on aging as planning and service areas.

The Area Agencies on Aging are local nonprofit agencies that contract with public and private organizations to provide services for older adults in their area. They are a vital resource for services and programs available for senior adults. Area Agencies on Aging go by a variety of names, such as Bureau on Aging, Council of Senior Services, Commission on the Elderly, or Center for Elder Affairs. These agencies can direct people to services in their neighborhood, send booklets and brochures on specific topics, and, in some cases, let them talk to a case manager who will discuss the needs of an older adult and refer them to or arrange for appropriate help. People can find their local Area Agency on Aging by calling the Eldercare Locator or by calling their state unit on aging.

Q 26.21   What is the difference between Medicare and Medicaid?

Medicare is the federal health insurance program for people age 65 and older (and certain disabled people younger than age 65). If a person is eligible for Social Security benefits (including disability benefits), he or she may apply for Medicare. Medicare has two basic parts: hospital insurance (Part A) and medical insurance (Part B).

- Medicare Part A covers hospitalization, hospice care, some skilled nursing care, and some home health care from a Medicare-certified home healthcare agency.
- Medicare Part B covers 80% of necessary medical services and equipment, including doctors' fees; physical, occupational, and speech therapies; durable medical equipment (such as hospital beds and wheelchairs); x-rays; and lab tests. Medicare covers only a small portion of the long-term care services people may need if they have a chronic illness or disability. Most importantly, it will not cover personal or custodial care or supportive services, such as a homemaker or Meals-on-Wheels.

For more information about Medicare Parts A and B, call toll free 800-633-4227 or go to www.medicare.gov.

Medicaid is federal- and state-funded medical assistance for low-income individuals of all ages. Services under Medicaid are free, but strict financial eligibility requirements may require people to reduce or "spend down" their assets, income, and savings to reach the eligibility level. Different asset and income levels apply, depending on whether people receive care at home or in a nursing facility. Requirements change each year, so individuals should check with their county department of job and family services for current state requirements, rules, and restrictions.

Support and Information

Q 26.22   Are there support groups for adult children caring for aging loved ones?

Yes. Many support groups exist that are disease specific, such as those offered via a person's local Alzheimer, multiple sclerosis, or Parkinson associations. In addition, some support groups exist that are not disease specific in nature. One such group is Children of Aging Parents. A list of support groups by state is available at www.caps4caregivers.org. The Eldercare Locator is another resource that can link people to local support groups.

People who share experiences of a particular disease or disability can offer support and understanding to each other as well as tips on coping. By joining a support group, individuals can benefit from meeting new people in a similar situation and offer and receive help and advice.

Q 26.23   Are there any good resources on the Internet to help me to understand and access services available for my aging parents?

The Internet has a wealth of information to offer. Some suggested caregiver support sites include
- www.caregiver.org: Family Caregiver Alliance
- www.nfcacares.org: National Family Caregivers Association
- www.caregiving.org: National Alliance for Caregiving
- www.care-givers.com: Empowering Caregivers, which offers support, chat rooms, and information
- www.caregiver.com: Site of *Today's Caregiver* magazine, which provides information and support for caregivers
- www.agingwithdignity.org: This site has resources for planning for the end of life.

Other helpful sites can be found via the AoA (www.aoa.gov). The AoA Web site offers links to state entities serving older adults.

References

American Association of Homes and Services for the Aging. (2005, June). *What kinds of services are available?* Retrieved September 2, 2005, from http://www.aahsa.org/consumer_info/how_to_choose/services_available.asp

Ohio State University Extension. (2002, February). *Personal profile.* Retrieved May 15, 2005, from http://ohioline.osu.edu/ss-fact/pdf/0169.pdf

Rubenson, E. (2000). *When aging parents can't live alone: A practical family guide.* Los Angeles: Lowell House.

Resources

AARP: www.aarp.org

Administration on Aging: www.aoa.gov

American Association of Homes and Services for the Aging: www.aahsa.org

Continuing Care Accreditation Commission: www.carf.org/aging

Medicare: www.medicare.gov

National Association of Professional Geriatric Care Managers: www.caremanager.org

U.S. Department of Health and Human Services Eldercare Locator: 800-677-1116; www.eldercare.gov

U.S. Social Security Administration: www.ssa.gov or www.socialsecurity.gov

Chapter 27
Retirement Issues

Christine A. Price, PhD, CFLE

Background

Q 27.1 How might my decision to retire affect my adjustment?

The most important thing is that a woman feels ownership of her decision to retire. Frequently, husbands or family members encourage women to retire because of the needs of others. When a woman retires because of outside influences rather than of her own accord, she may experience feelings of resentment or regret (Price, 1998). A woman who retires because she wants to retire will adjust more successfully.

Q 27.2 Are there stages of retirement that I can expect to encounter?

Retirement often is viewed as an "event." However, retirement is actually both a *process* (requiring planning and adjustment) and a *life stage* (lasting for multiple years). As a result of numerous research studies, Atchley (Atchley & Barush, 2004) developed six phases of retirement that represent a transitional process that individuals go through when they permanently exit the workforce. These phases are preretirement, retirement, disenchantment, reorientation, retirement routine, and termination of retirement. These phases do not apply to everyone, of course, because retirement is experienced on an individual basis. Furthermore, these stages were established primarily as a result of studies involving men. Researchers still are attempting to document the extent of gender differences that occur during retirement.

Q 27.3 What happens after the newness or "honeymoon period" of retirement wears off?

It is common for women (and men, for that matter) to experience some disenchantment with retirement once the newness has worn off. One can only golf or garden so many hours before that activity begins to lose its luster. Disenchantment may result from boredom or disappointment if a planned event or goal could not be realized. For those retirees who experience some feelings of dissatisfaction, it is important to set goals and to look for ways to be productive. Try to establish a schedule (whether strict or flexible) to provide a sense of purpose to each day.

Q 27.4   Do women who enter the workforce later in life (such as after raising their children) view retirement differently?

Women who establish a career later in adulthood sometimes do not feel ready for retirement. They may feel frustration that at the time they are achieving professional goals and feeling competent in their work, their spouse or other family members feel it is time for them to retire (Carp, 1997). For these women, retirement comes too soon. It is important to consider the retirement decision carefully. People must not make the mistake of sacrificing their own needs and goals based on the opinions of others.

Q 27.5   Why are retirement goals important?

Goals are important at any stage of life but are particularly important in retirement because they give people purpose, provide an opportunity for learning, and promote a sense of accomplishment. Goals in retirement also help to define who individuals are when work roles are no longer available. Retirement goals are personal and can vary widely based on individual abilities and interests. For example, one person's ambition might be to establish an exercise program, whereas someone else might aspire to learn a new language. Just because a person has retired does not mean she stops being productive or stops having a desire to learn and connect with the world around her. The goals people set in retirement and in later life in general help them maintain who they are and provide an avenue for growth (Vaillant, 2002).

Adjusting to Retirement

Q 27.6   Is it common for women to miss the social relationships they had in their former work roles?

Missing daily interactions with customers, colleagues, clients, and students often is an unexpected part of retirement. Whether in service-oriented roles or in leadership positions, women who are retiring today have worked in situations that involved interacting with others.

Following retirement, women, including married women, may experience feelings of loneliness. They feel disconnected despite their efforts to keep in touch with former work friends. Although they do not miss work, they often miss the people (Price, 1998).

 27.7   What can I do if I begin to feel lonely or isolated in retirement?

In retirement, it is critical for people to expand or develop a social network of friends and family with whom they can interact on a regular basis. Because retired women may no longer have daily contact with others, especially if they are single, they need to place a higher priority on maintaining social relationships than they might have in the past. Although it may be tempting to rely on family members for all of one's social needs, it is important to establish one's own circle of friends and acquaintances. Frequently, it is through new interests and activities that social relationships develop.

 27.8   I've been a nurse for many years. What happens to my identity when I am no longer practicing that nursing role every day?

For women who have worked outside of the home for many years, it is not uncommon to experience some feelings of loss related to the work role. For example, women may report feeling a loss of social status or of their professional identity when they retire. At the same time, many women have alternative social roles they fall back on in retirement, and these help to counter any identity crisis they may experience (Price, 2000, 2003). A way to handle this role change is for individuals to recognize other ways they identify themselves, for example, mother, friend, volunteer, or returning student. Rather than focus on the loss of the work role, they can emphasize the new roles that they now have more time to explore.

 27.9   After all of my years of nursing, I feel I have a lot to offer the next generation. How do I share my knowledge and experience?

The experiences and wisdom of retirees are assets often overlooked by the larger society as well as retirees. Fortunately, greater recognition is being placed on the importance of volunteers and the value of their contributions. A superb way for one to share her knowledge is through community volunteer work. Whether in a professional capacity or not, retirees have a great deal to offer the younger generation. For example, a retired nurse can serve as a mentor to nursing students and new nursing professionals, use her skills to care for chil-

dren or older adults, or serve as a hospice volunteer for families in
need. Retired nurses have unique value because of their healthcare
experience as well as their nurturing qualities. By utilizing their skills
in retirement, in whatever capacity they choose, they can continue to
feel productive and experience considerable fulfillment. (Remember
that retirees will need to maintain an active nursing license if they in-
tend to do any nursing work, even as a volunteer.)

**Q 27.10   I'm used to feeling challenged and stimulated by my work. How do
I keep my mind active after retirement?**

People can choose to view retirement as an ending or a beginning.
Those who approach retirement as an opportunity to grow and
learn, as well as relax and have fun, will continue to feel challenged
and stimulated by the world around them. Research consistently
has shown that being engaged in the world, whether through for-
mal education or informal activities, contributes positively to one's
health, well-being, and longevity (Vaillant, 2002). Lifelong learning
can be accomplished in a variety of ways—for example, learning an
instrument or language, reading a book, doing a crossword puzzle,
using a computer, practicing a favorite hobby, or taking continuing
education courses at a local university. Many universities encourage people older than the age of 60 to enroll in courses at no cost
except for purchasing textbooks or other course materials. Older
adults should check with colleges or universities in their area. Older
adults also can participate in Elderhostel, which is a not-for-profit
organization designed to provide learning adventures for people 55
and older. For more information about Elderhostel programs, go to
www.elderhostel.org. Learning also can involve taking on new roles
in retirement, such as teacher, mentor, or volunteer. The brain requires exercise to stay in shape. Retirees must make a concerted effort in retirement to learn new things, form new relationships, and
continue to grow to their full potential.

Family Relations

**Q 27.11   My husband and I are retiring next year. What can we do to ease the
transition into this new stage of our marriage?**

Retirement is a new stage in any marriage and requires careful ne-
gotiation. Research indicates that couples adjust more successfully
to retirement when both spouses retire at the same time. It is neces-

sary for retiring spouses to accomplish a few things related to goals, boundaries, and communication.

First, be sure to establish mutual retirement goals. When one spouse envisions retirement in an RV and the other in the garden, conflict or disappointment can result. Additionally, spouses need to think about goals or activities they plan to pursue independently of each other. Retirement is a great opportunity for spending more time together as a couple; however, it is equally important that spouses maintain their individual identities and friendship networks.

Second, having both husband and wife at home increases the potential for conflict. The most common topics for disagreement are the division of household tasks and personal space. Clearly outline which spouse is responsible for what, and avoid criticizing how tasks are completed.

Finally, good communication between spouses is the key to a happy retirement together. Spouses should talk openly about their feelings, goals, and concerns related to retirement as well as their relationship. Use this stage of the marriage as an opportunity to achieve greater intimacy and reestablish a lasting friendship.

Q 27.12 **My husband is retiring next year, but I have chosen to work a few more years to increase my pension income. What are some suggestions for this transition?**

This situation is often referred to as "dissynchronized" retirement and can result in reduced marital satisfaction for the working wife. The primary complaint of working wives with retired husbands is that the women still feel responsible for all of the household tasks and are not receiving assistance from their retired husbands. It is important that the couple agree on how to divide household duties and other responsibilities. Furthermore, for wives not to feel pressured to retire or feel frustrated by a husband who loafs around the house all day, it is important that the husband identifies what he is going to do with his time. Whether it is golf, fishing, part-time employment, or volunteering in the community, husbands need to have a retirement plan that does not depend on the input or involvement of their working wives (Yogev, 2002).

Q 27.13 **Do married women have a "better" retirement experience than single women?**

Overall, preliminary studies show that retired married women report higher retirement satisfaction levels than single women (Marks &

Lambert, 1998). This finding is attributed to the likelihood of having a higher income, being involved in family responsibilities, and having the companionship of a husband. At the same time, studies also are showing that married women are not as successful as single women at establishing and maintaining their own social support networks and friendships in retirement. Retired women who are divorced, widowed, or never married spend more time nurturing their social relationships and, in times of need, are able to call upon a number of people to provide emotional or instrumental support.

Q 27.14   My daughter seems to think that when I retire, I will become a full-time babysitter. Although I love my grandchildren and want to spend time with them, I also have other interests. How can I communicate my feelings without upsetting my daughter?

Historically, women have been socialized to nurture, provide care, and basically put the needs of others in front of their own. Although these practices are commendable and often necessary sacrifices, retirement is a time for women to finally consider their own desires and goals. Too often, women retire and fall into a caregiving role for aging parents, young grandchildren, or an ill relative without questioning whether this is what they want to do. In some circumstances, there is no one else to offer assistance, and retired women feel obligated to provide care. At the same time, retired women have the right and duty to themselves to establish boundaries in their families that provide them with time to pursue their own interests. To protect themselves, it is important for retirees to calmly but firmly outline what caregiving responsibilities they are comfortable with (if any at all). If family members do not understand or become upset, the retirees need to clearly repeat the boundaries they have established and stand firm. A balance between family responsibilities and personal growth in retirement is something all women deserve and should not instigate feelings of guilt.

Self-Care and Time Management

Q 27.15   My work as a nurse kept me on my feet and moving constantly. How do I stay healthy now that I've retired?

Paying attention to one's health and wellness is very important in retirement. Many ways exist to incorporate healthy living habits into retirement, but the first step is to have a complete physical exam with a healthcare provider. Find out what physical activity is appropriate. Even if individuals have never exercised regularly, retirement is an ideal opportunity to start! Women now have time to devote to their own needs, and nothing is more important than one's health. They should establish a regular exercise routine that they can enjoy and that fits into their schedule. For those who prefer to exercise with a companion, they can ask a friend or spouse to join them. Also, individuals need to pay attention to what they are eating and how the food they eat makes them feel. Do they have lots of energy? Are they eating too much sugar or drinking too much caffeine? Retirement is just the beginning of a new stage of life, so women should take this opportunity to start fresh! Remember, absolutely no truth exists to the myth that "you can't teach an old dog new tricks."

Q 27.16 **A friend of mine retired two years ago, and she seems busier than when she was working full time. I want to experience a fulfilling retirement, but how do I balance being active and having leisure time?**

A word of advice often shared by retired women is "Learn to say no!" This is an important tip, and one that newly retired women need to use. Despite expectations that retirement will be full of free time and personal autonomy, it is common for women to be approached immediately following their retirement by friends, family, community, and faith-based organizations to share their time (Price, 1998). Although being active and involved in retirement is a good thing, there can be too much of a good thing. It is critical that women, especially those recently retired, outline the amount of time they will contribute to others and the types of activities they want to do and then stick to this plan. Preserve time for relaxation and pleasure. They should only get involved in things that they really want to do. By learning to say no, they can take control of their retirement rather than have retirement control them.

Q 27.17 **I'm used to taking care of others. How do I take care of myself in retirement?**

It is important for retired women to approach this life stage as an opportunity to say "my turn!" Because women spend a considerable portion of their adult lives taking care of others and putting the needs of others first, retirement provides a chance to look inward and consider, possibly for the first time, their own needs and desires. This is not to suggest that retirement should be a time of complete self-absorption to the point of no responsibility. However, it can be a time for personal reflection and growth. To establish a balance between caring for others and caring for themselves, women need to set priorities and communicate these priorities to those around them. It often helps to include female friends in this process. Women can encourage each other to maintain this balance, look after each other, and provide a gentle reminder when one friend's self-care is getting pushed aside.

Q 27.18 How can I balance caregiving responsibilities for my spouse (or grandchildren or aging parent) with my own retirement goals?

First, a person in this situation should be commended for her recognition of the need for balance in her retirement. If women have family responsibilities that take a good deal of their time, it is important to outline a schedule that preserves time for their own interests, whether that means solitary relaxation, time to do a favorite hobby, or a chance to go out to lunch with a friend. Retirees should outline goals for themselves that are both short term and long term. What things give them pleasure? What are activities or interests that they never had time for? Maybe it is taking a trip, or maybe it is just to read an entire book. When an individual reaches a goal, celebrate! In addition to setting their own goals, retirees can utilize support from their family or community services. Often women feel as though they must be everything to everyone, which, of course, is an unrealistic expectation. Retired women should not feel guilty about asking for help or sharing caregiving responsibilities with others; they have earned this retirement. Besides, they will not be much help to their loved ones if they do not take proper care of themselves.

Q 27.19 I'm going to be living on a limited income once I retire. How can I have a fulfilling retirement experience without spending a lot of money?

Fortunately, feeling fulfilled emotionally or psychologically does not come with a price tag. Personal fulfillment is a subjective experience and can result from a variety of things unrelated to material possessions or activities associated with wealth. To experience a fulfilling retirement, individuals first have to identify what types of things give them pleasure. What things help them to feel productive or needed by others? What engages their interest and enthusiasm? Some suggestions that do not require a hefty bank account include

• **Volunteering:** People can consider volunteering in their community. Frequently, volunteers can set their own schedule and can choose the types of people they work with and activities they do. Every person has something to offer, and the act of giving to others will result in immeasurable rewards. Contact the local Retired and Senior Volunteer Program (RSVP, www.seniorcorps.org), which is part of Senior Corps—a network of national service programs that provides older Americans an opportunity to apply their life experience to meeting community needs. Those older than 55 are eligible to volunteer with RSVP in programs across the United States as well as in Puerto Rico and the Virgin Islands.

- **Lifelong learning:** Practice lifelong learning in retirement by reading books from the library, learning new things, or just being engaged with the world around oneself. Retirement is an opportunity for growth and development, which contributes to feelings of satisfaction and confidence. Older adults can challenge themselves to attend a class as part of an over-60 program, learn a new activity, or read a book—it is never too late to move in new directions!

- **Socializing with others:** Retirees can make new friends, contact old friends, and place themselves in social environments. Personal fulfillment can emerge from interactions with others in a variety of settings, including book clubs, the local senior center, or faith-based organizations. Relationships with others can significantly affect individuals' psychological and emotional well-being in later life. As a result, retirement is a time to rejuvenate old relationships and cultivate new ones.

Factors Affecting Retirement

Q 27.20   **How important are friendships for women in retirement?**

Friendships, particularly female friendships, are very important to women in retirement for a number of reasons. First, retirement sometimes results in a loss of social contact and regular interaction with others. Friendships fill that void and provide retired women with an important source of social support. Second, as any other life transition, retirement can involve both joys and challenges. Having friends to lean on and share with, especially other women having similar experiences, can be very satisfying. Third, because of differences in longevity, women are more likely than men to be widowed in retirement. Consequently, friendships in retirement supply a critical source of emotional support as well as instrumental assistance during the illness or death of a spouse. Finally, friendships help to validate who people are as well as provide access to alternative views and experiences. By having friends in retirement, individuals can continue to grow and feel engaged with those around them.

Q 27.21   Does race or ethnicity affect women's retirement experiences?

Unfortunately, not a great deal of research has been done that examines retirement differences among women from different racial/ethnic backgrounds. Cultural expectations surrounding women's work and family responsibilities likely influence how family members and women view the retirement transition. For example, in cultures where women do not traditionally work outside of the home, retirement may not be viewed as a woman's issue. On the other hand, in cultures where women have consistently worked outside of the home, the option of retiring would depend significantly on economic class. In lower socioeconomic groups, retirement may be viewed as a luxury and not an option for many women. What appears to have greater influence on women's retirement beyond race or ethnicity is income. Women from higher socioeconomic brackets are more likely to retire, whereas women with lower incomes may need to continue working. Other influential factors include employment history and marital status. Women with more investment in the work role have greater difficulty adjusting to retirement, and women who are married in retirement generally show higher retirement satisfaction (Price, 1998).

Q 27.22   I recently read that because people are living longer today, they can spend an average of 20–25 years in retirement. Is that true?

Yes, it is true. People today, both men and women, are healthier than ever before, and as a result, they are living longer. Life expectancy at the turn of the 20th century (1900) was 47 years. This number gradually increased to 68 years in 1950 and is 77 years today (Hetzel & Smith, 2001). This 30-year increase in longevity has resulted in a dramatic increase in the years people spend in retirement. Because women, on average, live six years longer than men, they can realistically spend 20 or more years in retirement. What was historically a brief stage of life (people died soon after retiring, if they quit working at all) has become a "third" stage of older adulthood, one that comes after "empty nest" and before being "elderly." One consequence of this increase in retirement years is the opportunity to spend more time pursuing personal interests and being with family. At the same time, however, people have a greater need to be financially prepared to live for an extended time on a limited income. Because of their discontinuous work histories, lack of pension eligibility, likelihood of being widowed, and risk of chronic health conditions in later life, women are at particular economic risk in retirement. As a result, women need to begin planning for their retirement early. They must not depend on their husbands to do the planning or assume that their husband's retirement income will be sufficient.

Q 27.23 Because women live, on average, longer than men, they are likely to be widowed in retirement. What are things women should do to put their affairs in good order?

Because women are more likely to experience widowhood in retirement, it is very important that married women are informed about the sources of their retirement income (such as a pension, Social Security, financial investments) and whether their annual income would change if their husbands die. They also need to know whether they have long-term care insurance, what outstanding debts or mortgages they are financially responsible for, and what end-of-life arrangements have been made for both themselves and their spouse. These are not popular topics of conversation, but they are critical to the security of retired women. Too frequently, women are not prepared or informed about their retirement and depend on their husbands to handle all retirement-related matters. Women need to be proactive and utilize available resources such as those listed at the end of this chapter to plan for their future in retirement.

Q 27.24 How can I be sure I am informed about issues that are critical to my welfare in retirement (e.g., savings and assets, insurance documentation, retirement income, long-term care resources)?

Women can find answers to these questions by talking openly with their spouse, their attorney, their healthcare provider, and/or other family members. They should be proactive and persistent in getting the information they need. Regardless of a woman's marital status, she must not be deterred if someone tells her, "Don't worry about those things." It is only through proper planning that women can ensure their own financial and physical security in retirement.

Q 27.25 Why don't we have more information about women's retirement?

The primary reason that such limited information exists about retirement and women is because for many years, it was assumed that women did not retire. Despite the fact that women have been working both inside and outside of the home for centuries, retirement was associated only with men. For women who work inside of the home, retirement often never takes place. Women's work continues in the home, caring for family members. For women who work outside of the home (in addition to inside the home), the retirement transition has become more relevant. As a result, researchers are taking a specific interest in examining women's retirement.

Q 27.26   How is retirement different for men as opposed to women?

A common misperception is that retirement for men and women is very much the same. For both men and women, retirement is something they often look forward to, a stage of life associated with relaxation and pleasure. However, because men and women have divergent work histories, have different social roles and family responsibilities, earn unequal salaries, and have different life expectancies, retirement can be quite different for men and women. For example, research indicates that women spend more years in retirement than men, experience the loss of social contacts more severely than men, often retire because of caregiving responsibilities, rarely qualify for pensions, and are more economically disadvantaged in retirement than men (Price, 1998). These differences can significantly affect women's emotional, psychological, and financial well-being in retirement. Because researchers' knowledge about women's retirement is still in the preliminary stages, investigators must continue to recognize the unique nature of women's retirement and work toward a more comprehensive understanding of this important and increasingly lengthy life stage.

References

Atchley, R.C., & Barush, A. (2004). *Social forces and aging* (10th ed.). Belmont, CA: Wadsworth.

Carp, F. (1997). Retirement and women. In J.M. Coyle (Ed.), *Handbook on women and aging* (pp. 112–128). Westport, CT: Greenwood Press.

Hetzel, L., & Smith, A. (2001). *The 65 years and over population: 2000* (Census 2000 brief C2KBR/01-10). Washington, DC: U.S. Department of Commerce, Economics and Statistics Administration, U.S. Census Bureau.

Marks, N., & Lambert, J.D. (1998). Marital status continuity and change among young and midlife adults. *Journal of Family Issues, 19,* 652–686.

Price, C.A. (1998). *Women and retirement: The unexplored transition.* New York: Garland.

Price, C.A. (2000). Women and retirement: Relinquishing professional identity. *Journal of Aging Studies, 14,* 81–101.

Price, C.A. (2003). Professional women's retirement adjustment: The experience of reestablishing order. *Journal of Aging Studies, 17,* 341–355.

Vaillant, G.E. (2002). *Aging well: Surprising guideposts to a happier life from the landmark Harvard study of adult development.* Boston: Little, Brown.

Yogev, S. (2002). *For better or for worse—but not for lunch: Making marriage work in retirement.* New York: Contemporary Books.

Resources

Administration on Aging: (www.aoa.gov) see the "Money Matters" link in the "Elders and Families" section.

American Savings Education Council: www.asec.org

Bauer-Maglin, N., & Radosh, A. (Eds.). (2003). *Women confronting retirement: A nontraditional guide.* New Brunswick, NJ: Rutgers University Press.

Financial Security in Later Life: www.csrees.usda.gov/nea/economics/fsll/fsll.html see the link "Tools for Consumers."

Social Security Administration: www.ssa.gov; content designed specifically to address women's Social Security issues can be located at www.ssa.gov/women

Women's Institute for a Secure Retirement: www.wiser.heinz.org

Index

The letter t after page number indicates that relevant content appears in a table.

12-step programs, 174–175

A

AARP, 254, 257
abdominal breathing, 227–228
absentmindedness. *See* memory loss
abuse. *See* domestic violence
achlorhydria, 181
acquired immune deficiency syndrome (AIDS), 114–115, 119
ACTH. *See* adrenocorticotropin
active ingredients, in herbal supplements, 197–198
adaptogens, 198, 210
Administration on Aging (AoA), 278–280, 293
adrenal exhaustion, 209
adrenal glands, 224
adrenaline, 224
adrenocorticotropin (ACTH), 224
adult day care/service, 270, 273
advance directives, 275–276
African American women, heart disease risk in, 2
Agency for Healthcare Research and Quality, 144
aging
   and bone mineral density, 14
   and breast cancer risk, 26
   and uterine cancer risk, 50
aging parents, 255–256, 267–269. *See also* older adults
   caring for, 269–271, 288
   housing options for, 272–273
   relationship with, 255–256

support groups, 279–280
AIDS. *See* acquired immune deficiency syndrome
airline flights, lymphedema risk from, 34
Al-Anon/Alateen, 172–173, 175
alcohol consumption. *See also* chemical dependency
   bone loss from, 20, 182
   and tattooing/body piercing, 123
   urinary incontinence from, 84
Alcoholics Anonymous, 175
alcoholism, signs/symptoms of, 171. *See also* chemical dependency
alendronate (Fosamax®), for osteoporosis treatment, 17
allodynia, 71
alpha-fetoprotein, 52
Alzheimer's Association, 270
American Association of Homes and Services for the Aging (AAHSA), 272–273, 280
American Association of Naturopathic Physicians, 211
American Cancer Society, 43, 55, 68, 143t, 220
American College of Obstetricians and Gynecologists, 192
American College of Rheumatology (ACR), fibromyalgia diagnosis criteria of, 69
American Dietetic Association, 188
American Heart Association, 10, 143t
American Joint Committee on Cancer, staging criteria of, 61–62
American Lung Association, 143t
American Nurses Association, 177, 254
American Savings Education Council, 293
American Social Health Association (ASHA), 110, 119

E

F